NINJA FOODI

PRESSURE COOKER

365 DAYS OF QUICK, EASY & DELICIOUS RECIPES FOR YOUR NEW NINJA FOODI AIR FRYER AND PRESSURE COOKER

BY GREG MASON

TABLE OF CONTENTS

CHAPTER 1
INTRODUCTION

ENTER THE FOODI

I know the struggle. If you're holding this book right now, you know the same feeling all too well. Trying to decide what to put on the table, be it for yourself, for family, or for your closest friends can be stressful to say the least. But we all eat 3 times a day, so why not make things a bit more streamlined? Why not make the entire process easier, simpler, and faster? And why not make all of these meals in one pot instead of using the dozen other kitchen utensils that tend to clutter out kitchen drawers? Enter the Ninja Foodi - your new best friend - and me, here to assist you along this path to absolutely delicious food that pretty much cooks itself.

As a professional chef and former recipe developer for a large number of Michelin star restaurants, you may wonder why I am here telling you to go out and buy yet another trendy, all-in-one kitchen gadget. Well, let me tell you... it's because I've seen what the Ninja Foodi is capable of. And to say I have been impressed would be quite the understatement. I've literally seen it transform people's entire cooking experience, making it simpler, better, faster, far more pleasant and mouth wateringly delicious. I've also put this device through its paces, often using it for almost every dish for full blown dinner parties of 12. You will soon discover how, at the push of a button (or maybe two), you will be able to take all of the work out of getting that sumptuous meal on the table in the blink of an eye. This nifty appliance can bake, air crisp/air fry, roast, broil, pressure cook, and slow cook. You may want to read that again.

It's truly in another league when comparing it to other counter-top appliances, both the way it performs and the unique style that it has, not to mention its high-quality build. It replaces your multi-cooker, slow cooker, pressure cooker, and your air fryer - all with one multi use, singular pot. Now I'm not saying the Ninja Foodi will replace your entire kitchen, but boy, does it come really close. In fact, I developed every recipe in this book while road tripping across the country with my husband in a smaller-than-average RV! Who needs a full-size kitchen when you have the Foodi by your side? All I took with me on the trip was a knife, small cutting board, a few bowls and my trusty Ninja Foodi. I did my absolute best not to use any other special equipment like blenders or other appliances in this book, and if I did it's always completely optional, not mandatory. Ready to learn more? Let's dive right in!

GETTING TO KNOW THE FOODI'S FUNCTIONS

There are more than just a few things that the Foodi is great at: pressure cooking tougher proteins into tender, fall-off-the-bone scrumptiousness? Check. Crisping veggies and proper baked desserts? Double check. Deep frying a whole turkey? Um, I wouldn't recommend it, but worth a try!
When I started to come up with ideas for recipes included in this book, I made sure I laid out a few key ground rules. For one, I wanted all of the ingredients included to be accessible. How did I achieve this? Most of the shopping for this book was done at either Walmart or Target. No hard to find specialty ingredients found in this book, since I was in an RV and it would be near impossible to get my hands on any anyway! Let me emphasize, I wanted this book to be simple and easy. You'll see that I uphold my word, since no other electrical devices are used to make and recipes in this book.

I depended solely on the Foodi for many months on end - no oven, no microwave, no nada. This single pointed use made me an expert with the appliance in a very short time. Here are the five things you need to know about how the Foodi cooks:

1. It applies heat from the bottom
2. It applies heat from the top
3. Then it circulates heat via its high-powered fan
4. Then applies pressure when the Pressure Lid is locked into place
5. Last but not least, it keeps time.

The true magic occurs when you know exactly how to use these things in conjunction with one another. Broiling, for example, is nothing more than heating from the upper portion of the Foodi at its maximum heat. Pressure cooking is heating from the bottom, all while the Pressure Lid is locked in its place. Air crisping (also known as Air Frying) is cooking at high heat with the fan on to circulate it equally around the food. Here are some specifics about the different ways of cooking and settings on the Foodi.

Pressure:
The Foodi can cook food very quickly while under pressure. Dried beans can literally take a fraction of the time when compared to normal cooking, and the same goes for chicken stock. In order to do this, all you need is to put the food and liquid called for into the inner pot, lock the Pressure Lid, set the valve to Seal, and then set the timer to bring the pressure up in the Foodi. When you see the red safety valve pop up in its tallest position you know the Foodi is at its maximum pressure. Once the timer automatically turns the Foodi off, you can either quick release the built up pressure by moving the valve to the "VENTING" position and very carefully remove the lid , or alternatively you can let the pressure release naturally by waiting until the red safety valve lowers all the way down with time, then remove the lid afterword.

In many recipes I will instruct you to naturally release the pressure after cooking and then ask to turn the Foodi off. Reason being, the "Keep Warm" setting kicks in automatically upon completion of the pressure cooking. This is one of the many safety features, but the "Keep Warm" function delays the natural release of pressure. And sometimes this slow release of pressure is exactly what we are looking for.

Never pressure-cooked before? Allow me to explain what exactly happens in the pot. Once heated to a certain temperature (around 212 degrees), the liquids in the pot turn to gas. As we know from grade school science, gas can be compressed- whereas liquid cannot. This gas is trapped in the pot while the liquid continues to turn into gas, and voilà - pressure is formed. That pressure forces flavor and aroma compounds into the food being cooked– at a microscopic level. To appreciate the beauty of this process, think of the following: if you pressure cook a chicken breast in lemony flavored water, even if the chicken doesn't ever touch the water, it have a lemon zesty taste. This is due to the fact that the pressure has forced the lemon flavor directly into the chicken - again, at a microscopic level. It works twofold as pressure also builds up heat. As mentioned before, liquids evaporate at 212°F, but because of this very High pressure inside the Foodi the temperature can easily reach around 240°F. It's basically the opposite of what happens when cooking at higher altitudes with lower atmospheric pressure – where water boils at a much lower temperature. This time it boils at much higher.

Steam Setting
Used for circulating steam in order to cook the food, this setting is for a gentler way of cooking, which many people believe to be one of the healthiest. Steaming is great for veggies and fish, but a steamed steak is not something I would recommend. To utilize the "Steam" function, lock on the Pressure Lid but leave it in the "vented" position, allowing the steam to freely escape through the valve and never reach high pressure.

Slow Cook
The slow cook function is admittedly the one I use the least, as I prefer to pressure cook instead. If you are looking to make something in the morning and enjoy it that evening, slow cooking would be the way to go. The Foodi will be heating from the bottom element with this function, but only with enough heat to bring the liquid to a slow boil. Excellent for making collagen rich bone broths and hearty, flavorful stews. Can take a long time, but is worth the wait in the end.

Air Crisp

This is convection cooking at its finest. The Air Crisp function has the fan operating at its highest speed. To really get a feel for just how great this is, try cooking up some pizza rolls on the default setting and compare it to your own oven afterwards. What you'll find is that in the Foodi there's no need to preheat the oven and no need to flip the rolls over for even baking. That's all thanks to the fan, which is at its maximum speed, circulating the air evenly while this function is engaged.

Saute/Sear

Functioning nearly the same as heating a skillet on a stovetop, the Sauté/Sear function is what you'll be using to do most of your "basic" day to day cooking. Remember to always preheat when using this function. Similarly, to a regular skillet atop a burner or electric stove top, the heat does not transfer instantaneously.

Bake/Roast

This function allows the Foodi to run its fan at the lowest speed, so as not to upset your fragile baked goods with its whirlwind-like forces.

Broil

This is the hottest setting on the Foodi. Browning and toasting has never been easier, and is best on the Broil function. It is far less temperamental than the broiler in your standard oven, so I trust it with all of my dishes that require broiling.

Keep Warm

A very useful function for keeping your food around 160°F. An example of this would be if you made tacos, wrapped them in foil, and placed them in the Foodi on the "Keep Warm" setting. You would have hot tacos to serve up any time. It comes in handy more than you would think, and I find myself using this function more frequently than I thought I would.

Setting the Temperature

The Foodi is flexible in that, once you've selected a function in the temperature range that you desire, you are able to adjust that temperature up and down as desired, as opposed to only using the default temperature setting for that function. The default for Air Crisping is set to 390°F, which is a great starting temperature to use while convection cooking.Whoever can up with this temperature is a genius, as your food will always turn out crispy-delicious-consistently. The main reason our friends over at Ninja included the ability to manually adjust the temperature is so that you can get creative with your own recipes and find sweet spots for the unique meals you make.

Setting the Time

Pressure-cooking, steaming, baking/roasting, slow-cooking, and dehydrating is controlled by the Foodi's built-in timer. It will cook for the time that you set it, and slowly decrease the heat and pressure intelligently, according to the function. Once the timer reaches zero, the Foodi will automatically activate the "Keep Warm" setting. There is no timer for searing and sautéing function because the manufacturers encourage you to cook using the visual cues of the food rather than to set cooking times.

USING AND MAINTAINING THE TOOLS

The Inner Pot

The interior of the Foodi's pot is lined with a thick nonstick ceramic coating and is made from high quality aluminum. This is the real workhorse of your Foodi, and you can do anything from making soups, to baking galettes and even searing fresh scallops. My recommendation is to buy an extra inner pot, as it often comes in handy when you are wanting to cook multiple things and eat at a later time. For those meal preppers out there, this is a must.

Although the aluminum shell is sturdy, the inner ceramic coating can scratch should you use abrasive materials with like steel tongs on it. This is why you should always use wooden or silicone-coated spatulas, tongs, spoons and other utensils when cooking in your Foodi. Having a pair of silicone mittens for your fingers (aka fittens) really come in handy when lifting the ultra-hot pot out of the Foodi base. You can usually pick them up off Amazon for under 5 dollars.

The Crisping Basket and Diffuser

These two nifty tools are designed to sit inside of the Foodi's inner pot. The Crisping basket is perforated with multiple openings, this is so that the heated air can easily circulate around the food when the fan is on. I occasionally use the crisping basket and diffuser in a way that they weren't actually intended. An example of this is that the crisping basket makes really lovely patterns for confectioners' sugar on baked recipes, and the diffuser is also able to hold large proteins in place while cooking - which I often use when cooking ribs.

Racks

Two racks are included with the Foodi. The smaller rack fits inside the crisper basket. This makes it possible to air crisp two items at once, just like baking two sheets of cookies on two different oven racks at the same time except there is no need to rotate the food since the air circulates around it. The second rack is conveniently reversible. It folds up for storage with ease and because it's reversible you are able to get the food much closer to the heating element for ultra-hot broiling. Using the reversible rack, you can fold the legs to make a table (what I like to call the "high position") which elevates the cooking food so it is extremely close to the top heating element, ideal for the most intense broiling. Similarly, to the smaller rack it also allows you to cook multiple things simultaneously. I like to cook my veggie or starches in the inner pot, with my proteins broiling on the rack in the "high" position at the top of the Foodi. With the legs reversed in the low position, it is able to hold various inserts, such as a springform pan or doughnut molds and also allows for steaming of foods without having it in direct contact with the liquid at the bottom of the pot.

Pressure Lid

 The final tool in your arsenal is the Pressure Lid. This is what's used whenever you want to Pressure Cook, Steam, or Slow Cook. Flip the pressure lid over and you will notice the underside contains a flexible plastic sealing ring which extends all the way around the outside edge. This is quite possibly the most important part of the lid, as it is what creates the all-important airtight seal between the lid and the base- which in turn allows the pressure to rapidly build during cooking. No seal means no pressure and food will just boil rather than being cooked under the pressure of the evaporated steam. I recommend checking that the sealing ring is free of particulate often, and also make sure it's in the corrected position before setting the Pressure Lid on top to prevent any leakages. After lots of use, normal wear and tear will occur and it may become slightly loose-fitting. I always have a backup at handy, just in case this happens. Without the sealing ring, it's impossible to cook under pressure.

The other two small outcroppings on the underside of the Pressure Lid are valves. The left valve controls the locking mechanism. If enough pressure is present to push this valve up, the lid locks automatically, ensuring your safety. The other valve was created to keep the food particles from spewing out of the pressure when you quick-release the pressure. This can be removed by cleaning, as starches can clog it.

To the right-hand side is the red safety valve. When this one pops up, the pot is under high pressure. This red safety valve will only pot up when the Foodi is set to the "Seal" position.

Now that we understand all the basics of the Ninja Foodi, it's time for the fun part: FOOD! Get your apron ready and let's get cooking!

CHAPTER 2
BREAKFASTS

CREAMY MANGO OATS

COOKING TIME: 10 MIN | SERVES 4

INGREDIENTS:

- 1 cup steel-cut oats
- 4 allspice berries
- ½ tsp. salt
- ½ cup whole milk
- 2 tbsp. brown sugar, light
- 1/4 cup kiwi, sliced
- 1/4 cup mango, sliced
- 1/4 cup banana, sliced
- Toasted coconut (to garnish)

Directions:

1. Add allspices, 3 cups water, salt, and oats to the inner pot of the Ninja Foodi Cooker.
2. Put on its lid, lock it, and turn the pressure handle to the SEAL position.
3. Select Pressure Cook mode, set the pressure to High, and cooking time to 10 minutes. Hit the START/STOP button to initiate cooking.
4. Once the oats are done, leave the cooker for 15 minutes to release the pressure naturally.
5. Quick-release the remaining pressure, then remove the lid of the Ninja Foodi cooker.
6. Remove and discard all the allspice berries.
7. Add brown sugar and milk to the oats.
8. Mix well, then serve with kiwi, mango, banana, and toasted coconuts on top.
9. Serve.

SOUR CREAM & CHIVES EGG SCRAMBLE

COOKING TIME: 9 MIN | SERVES 2

INGREDIENTS:

- 6 eggs, beaten
- 1 tbsp. sour cream
- 3 tbsp. cold butter, finely chopped
- ½ tsp. salt
- Cooking spray
- 1 tbsp. lemon juice
- Black pepper, to taste
- Chopped chives (to garnish)

DIRECTIONS:

1. Beat all the eggs with salt and butter in a suitable oil.
2. Grease the Ninja Foodi's cooking pot with cooking spray and place the Crisping Lid.
3. Select AIR CRISP mode, set the temperature to 390°F, and cooking time to 9 minutes. Hit the START/STOP button to initiate preheating.
4. After 1 minute, remove the lid and pour the egg mixture into the Ninja Foodi.
5. Cover the lid again and resume cooking until the machine beeps.
6. Remove its lid and add sour cream.
7. Garnish with black pepper, chives, and lemon wedges.
8. Enjoy.

CRIMINI BREADED CASSEROLE

COOKING TIME: 18 MIN | SERVES 4

INGREDIENTS:

- 1 tbsp. butter
- 2 medium shallots, minced
- 8 ounces crimini mushrooms, sliced
- 1 tsp. thyme leaves, minced
- 1 cup baby spinach leaves, torn
- ½ tsp. salt
- Black pepper, to taste
- 1 tbsp. plus 1 tsp. chives, chopped
- 4 eggs
- 4 Swiss cheese slices
- 1 baguette, sliced
- Zest of ½ lemon
- Cooking spray

Directions:

1. Select Sear/Sauté mode on the Ninja Foodi and add butter to its cooking pot.
2. When the butter is melted and lightly bubbling, add shallots and sauté for 3 minutes.
3. Add thyme, and mushrooms then sauté for 7 minutes.
4. Stir in spinach leaves and saute for 1 minute, then add 1 tbsp. chives, salt, and black pepper.
5. Divide this mushroom mixture into 4- 8 ounces ramekins.
6. Crack one egg into each ramekin while keeping the egg yolks intact.
7. Empty the Ninja Foodi's inner pot and fill it with ½ cup water.
8. Place the reversible rack in the pot and set the ramekins on this rack.
9. Put on the lid, lock it, and turn the pressure handle to the SEAL position.
10. Select Pressure Cook mode, set the pressure to LOW, and cooking time to 3 minutes. Hit the START/STOP button to initiate cooking.
11. Once done, release the pressure with a quick release, then remove the lid.
12. Grease the baguette slices with cooking spray.
13. Place a cheese slice and a baguette slice on top of each ramekin.
14. Return the ramekins to the cooking pot and put on the Crisping Lid.
15. Select Broil mode, and cooking time to 5 minutes. Hit the START/STOP button to initiate cooking.
16. Garnish the ramekins with lemon zest and chives.
17. Serve warm.

HAM & ARUGULA STUFFED OMELET

COOKING TIME: 5 MIN | SERVES 2

INGREDIENTS:

- 1 tbsp. butter, unsalted
- 6 eggs
- ½ tsp. salt
- 1/4 Cup Arugula
- 1/8 Deli ham
- 1/8 Feta, crumbled
- Chives (to garnish)
- Black pepper, to taste (to garnish)

DIRECTIONS:

1. Beat all six eggs with salt and black pepper in a bowl.
2. Select Sear/Sauté mode with Medium Heat on your Ninja Foodi.
3. Add unsalted butter to the inner pot and let it melt.
4. Pour in eggs mixture and cook for 2 minutes, put on the Crisping Lid
5. Select Air Crisp mode, set the temperature to 390°F and cooking time to 3 minutes. Hit the START/STOP button to initiate cooking.
6. Turn off and add ham, feta and arugula.
7. Fold and transfer the cooked omelet to a plate and garnish with black pepper and chives.
8. Enjoy.

CRUSTED BACON TART

COOKING TIME: 40 MIN | SERVES 9

INGREDIENTS:

- 1 (9-inch) frozen pie shell
- 6 eggs
- ½ cup heavy cream
- Salt, to taste
- Black pepper, to taste
- 1 cup Gruyère cheese, grated
- 1 cup bacon, cooked and crumbled

Directions:

1. Set the piecrust at room temperature for 15 minutes, then prick it with a fork.
2. Place the thawed crust in the lower portion of the Ninja Foodi's reversible rack.
3. Transfer this rack to the Ninja's inner pot and cover the Crisping Lid.
4. Select Bake/Roast mode, set the cooking time to 375°F, and cooking time to 10 minutes. Hit the START/STOP button to initiate cooking.
5. Once the crust is parbaked, remove the lid and transfer the crust to a pie plate.
6. Beat eggs with cream, salt, black pepper, cheese, and bacon in a bowl.
7. Pour this egg-cream mixture into the pie plate on top of the crust.
8. Return the crust to the reversible rack inside the Ninja food and cover the Crisping Lid.
9. Select Bake/Roast mode, set the temperature to 325°F, and cooking time to 30 minutes. Hit the START/STOP button to initiate cooking.
10. Once done, remove the lid and remove the quiche from the rack.
11. Allow it cool at room temperature, then slice.
12. Serve warm.

PANCAKES WITH BERRIES & CREAM

COOKING TIME: 16 MIN | SERVES 4

INGREDIENTS:

- ¾ cup whole milk
- 3 eggs
- 1 tsp. vanilla extract
- 4 tbsp. butter, melted
- ½ cup all-purpose flour
- 2 tbsp. cornstarch
- 1 tbsp. granulated sugar
- Whipped cream (to garnish)
- Assorted berries (to garnish)
- Confectioners' sugar (to garnish)

DIRECTIONS:

1. Beat all 3 eggs with milk in a mixing bowl for 1 minute until frothy.
2. Stir in 2 tbsp. butter and vanilla, then mix well.
3. Add granulated sugar, cornstarch and flour, then whisk until it makes a smooth batter.
4. Preheat the Ninja Foodi cooker on Sear/Sauté mode with High temperature for 5 minutes.
5. Once preheated, add butter and cook for 6 minutes with constant stirring.
6. Pour the pancake batter into the Ninja Foodi's pot and let it cook for 5minutes.
7. Put on the Crisping Lid, then select Bake/Roast mode, set the temperature to 375°F, and cooking time to 5 minutes. Hit the START/STOP button to initiate cooking.
8. Once the pancake is done, lift its lid and remove the cooking pot from the Ninja cooker.
9. Run a silicon spatula around the edges of the pancake and flip the pot on top of a serving plate to transfer the pancake.
10. Garnish with berries, whipped cream, and confectioners' sugar.
11. Enjoy.

BREAKFAST SPONGECAKE

COOKING TIME: 22 MIN | SERVES 4

INGREDIENTS:

- 2 cups all-purpose flour
- 3 tbsp. granulated sugar
- 2 tsp. baking powder
- ½ tsp. baking soda
- ½ tsp. salt
- 1½ cups whole milk
- 1 large egg
- 1 tbsp. fresh lemon juice
- 4 tbsp. butter, melted
- Cooking spray
- Confectioners' sugar
- Cocoa powder,
- Warm maple syrup

Directions:

1. Whisk flour with baking powder, granulated sugar, baking soda, and salt in a medium bowl.
2. Beat egg with lemon juice, milk, and melted butter in another medium bowl.
3. Gradually stir in all-purpose flour mixture and continue mixing until the batter is smooth.
4. Grease the Ninja Foodi's inner pot with cooking spray.
5. Pour the prepared batter into its pot and put on the Pressure Lid.
6. Lock the lid and turn the pressure handle to the SEAL position
7. Select Pressure Cook mode, set the pressure to Low and cooking time to 7 minutes. Hit the START/STOP button to initiate cooking.
8. Once it is done, replace the Pressure Lid with Crisping Lid.
9. Select Air Crisp mode, set the temperature to 390°F and cooking time to 15 minutes. Hit the START/STOP button to initiate cooking.
10. As the pancake cooks, spray its top with cooking spray after every 5 minutes.
11. When it's done, remove the inner pot from the Ninja Foodi and run a spatula around the cake.
12. Transfer the pancake to a platter and garnish with maple syrup, butter, and confectioner's sugar.
13. Slice and serve.

OLD-FASHOINED APPLE OATMEAL

COOKING TIME: 20 MIN | SERVES 8

INGREDIENTS:

- 2 cups old fashioned oatmeal
- 4 cups of water
- 3 tsp. cinnamon (ground)
- ½ cup heavy cream
- 3/4 cup dark brown sugar
- 1 ½ cups granny smith apples, sliced
- ½ tsp. of sea salt

DIRECTIONS:

1. Mix 4 cups water, oats, 2 tsp. cinnamon, salt, and ½ dark brown sugar in the Ninja Foodi's inner pot.
2. Put on the Pressure Lid and turn its pressure handle to the SEAL position.
3. Select Pressure Cook mode, set the pressure to LOW, and cooking time to 5 minutes. Hit the START/STOP button to initiate cooking.
4. Once it's done, release the pressure through a quick-release then remove the lid.
5. Mix remaining cinnamon and sugar with sliced apples in a bowl.
6. Add cream and apples to the oats and mix gently.
7. Again, put on the Pressure Lid and seal it.
8. Select Bake/Roast mode, set the temperature to 390°F, and cooking time to 15 minutes. Hit the START/STOP button to initiate cooking.
9. Once it's done, remove the lid.
10. Serve warm.

TOMATO SHAKSHUKA

COOKING TIME: 18 MIN | SERVES 6

INGREDIENTS:

- 2 red bell peppers, seeded, ribbed, and diced
- ½ medium yellow onion, diced
- 2 garlic cloves, minced
- 1 tbsp. tomato paste
- 1 (28-ounce) can crushed tomatoes
- 2 tbsp. Harissa
- 2 tsp. cumin ground
- ¼ cup olive oil
- ½ tsp. salt
- 6 eggs
- Pita bread (to garnish)

Directions:

1. Mix bell peppers with tomato paste, onion, crushed tomatoes, cumin, harissa, ½ cup water, and olive oil in the Ninja Foodi's inner pot.
2. Put on the Pressure Lid and turn the pressure handle to the SEAL position.
3. Select Pressure Cook mode, set the pressure to High and cooking time to 5 minutes. Hit the START/STOP button to initiate cooking.
4. Once done, release the pressure quickly, then remove the lid.
5. Switch the Ninja Foodi to Sear/Sauté mode on High heat, then sauté for 5 minutes.
6. Add salt to adjust seasoning, then mix well.
7. Make six wells in the tomato's mixture and crack one egg into each well.
8. Put on the Crisping Lid and cook on Broil mode for 8 minutes.
9. Serve warm with pita bread.

SPICED CHICKPEA SCRAMBLE

COOKING TIME: 12 MIN | SERVES 4

INGREDIENTS:

- 3 tbsp. peanut oil
- ½ medium yellow onion, diced
- 1 garlic clove, minced
- 8 ounces button mushrooms, sliced
- 1 cup cauliflower, chopped
- 2 tsp. cumin (ground)
- 2 tsp. turmeric (ground)
- 1 cup canned fire-roasted tomatoes, diced and drained
- 1 (14- to 16-ounce) block firm tofu, drained and crumbled
- 1 cup baby spinach leaves
- 1 cup canned chickpeas, drained
- 2 tsp. salt
- ground black pepper, to taste

DIRECTIONS:

1. Preheat your Ninja Foodi on Sear/Sauté mode at High temperature for 4 minutes.
2. Once preheated, toss in onion and garlic, then sauté for 3 minutes.
3. Stir in mushrooms and continue sautéing for 3 minutes.
4. Add turmeric, cumin, and cauliflower, then sauté for 2 minutes.
5. Stir in crumbled tofu and tomatoes, then put on the Pressure Lid.
6. Lock the lid and turn its pressure handle to the SEAL position.
7. Select Pressure Cook Mode, set the pressure to High, and set the time to 0 minutes.
8. When the machine beeps, release the pressure quickly, then remove the lid.
9. Toss in chickpeas and spinach and mix well.
10. Add black pepper and salt for seasoning, then mix again.
11. Serve warm.

SAVORY PORK PATTIES

COOKING TIME: 20 MIN | SERVES 6

INGREDIENTS:

- 1-pound ground pork
- 2 garlic cloves, minced
- 2 tsp. sage leaves, minced
- 1 tsp. maple syrup
- 1 tsp. red pepper flakes
- 1 tsp. salt
- ¼ tsp. ground black pepper
- Cooking spray

Directions:

1. Mix ground pork with garlic, sage, maple syrup, red pepper flakes, salt, and black pepper in a medium bowl.
2. Make 6 (1/2 inch) thick patties out of this pork mixture.
3. Place the Crisping Basket in the Ninja Foodi's inner port.
4. Grease the basket with a cooking spray and arrange the patties vertically in the basket.
5. Put on the Crisping Lid, then select Air Crisp mode, set the temperature to 390°F, and cooking time to 15 minutes. Hit the START/STOP button to initiate cooking.
6. Once the patties are cooked halfway through, remove the Crisping Lid, and arrange the patties in the basket horizontally then resume cooking.
7. Switch the Ninja Foodi to Broil mode and cook for 5 minutes.
8. Serve warm.

CHILI KALE EGG DISH

COOKING TIME: 22 MIN | SERVES 6

INGREDIENTS:

- 3 tbsp. peanut oil
- 1 medium yellow onion, diced
- 4 garlic cloves, minced
- 1 green bell pepper, seeded, and diced
- 2 serrano chiles, seeded, and diced
- 1 jalapeño, seeded, and diced
- 1 tbsp. cumin ground
- 1 tbsp. coriander ground
- 8 oz. kale leaves, finely chopped
- 1 tsp. salt
- 6 eggs
- Juice of ½ lemon
- 1 bunch cilantro leaves, chopped
- 2 tbsp. crumbled feta cheese
- 1 tbsp. finely chopped fresh dill

Directions:

1. Add oil, onion, garlic, bell pepper, and jalapeno to the Ninja Foodi's inner pot.
2. Select Sear/Sauté mode on high and sauté for 6 minutes.
3. Stir in coriander and cumin, then sauté for 3 minutes.
4. Add kale, then put on the Pressure Lid and turn the pressure handle to SEAL position.
5. Select Pressure Cook mode, set the pressure to High and cooking time to 5 minutes. Hit the START/STOP button to initiate cooking.
6. Once done, release the pressure quickly, then remove the lid.
7. Stir in cilantro, lemon juice, and salt.
8. Make 6 wells in the kale mixture and crack one egg into each well, then put on the Crisping Lid.
9. Select Air Crisp mode, set the temperature to 390°F and cooking time to 8 minutes. Hit the START/STOP button to initiate cooking.
10. Once done, garnish with shakshuka with dill and feta.
11. Serve warm.

CRISPY HASH BROWNS

COOKING TIME: 30 MIN | SERVES 10

INGREDIENTS:

- 4 medium russet potatoes, peeled and grated
- 2 tbsp. unsalted butter
- ¼ cup flour
- 1 tbsp. salt
- Black pepper, to taste
- Cooking spray

DIRECTIONS:

1. Soak grated potatoes in a bowl filled with water for 1 hour.
2. Transfer the potatoes to a cheesecloth and squeeze all the excess water out.
3. Preheat the Ninja Foodi on Sear/Sauté Mode on High.
4. Stir in Butter and potatoes, then sauté for 10 minutes.
5. Transfer the buttery potatoes to a bowl and add black pepper, salt, and flour. Mix well.
6. Layer a sheet pan with parchment paper.
7. Spread 1 cup of potato mixture on a plastic wrap and press it into a rectangular patty.
8. Repeat the same steps to make 10 patties and refrigerate them for 3 hours.
9. Transfer the patties to the Crisping basket and set the basket inside the Ninja Foodi's pot.
10. Put on the Crisping Lid, select Air Crisp mode set the temperature to 390°F and cooking time to 20 minutes. Hit the START/STOP button to initiate cooking.
11. Once done, remove the lid and serve the hash browns.
12. Enjoy.

PAPRIKA POTATOES HASH

COOKING TIME: 29 MIN | SERVES 6

INGREDIENTS:

- 3 pounds baby red potatoes
- 1 tbsp. 1 tsp. salt
- Cooking spray
- 1 tbsp. sweet paprika
- Black pepper, to taste

DIRECTIONS:

1. Add potatoes to the crisping basket and set this basket in the Ninja Foodi's inner pot.
2. Pour 1 cup water into the pot and drizzle 1 tbsp. salt over the potatoes.
3. Put on the Pressure Lid and turn the pressure handle to the SEAL position.
4. Select Pressure Cook mode, set the pressure to High and cooking time to 4 minutes. Hit the START/STOP button to initiate cooking.
5. Once done, remove the basket from the inner pot and discard the water.
6. Return the potatoes in the basket to the pot and spray them with cooking spray.
7. Drizzle remaining salt and black pepper over the potatoes.
8. Put the Crisping Lid, select Air Crisp mode, set the temperature to 390°F, and cooking time to 25 minutes. Hit the START/STOP button to initiate cooking.
9. Toss the potatoes after every 5 minutes.
10. Serve warm.

SHIITAKE CHILI CASSEROLE

COOKING TIME: 38 MIN | SERVES 4

INGREDIENTS:

Sauce
- ½ cup gochujang paste
- ¼ cup hard apple cider
- 1 tbsp. maple syrup
- 2 tsp. apple cider vinegar
- 1 tsp. toasted sesame oil
- ½ tsp. cinnamon ground

Casserole
- 6 tbsp. peanut oil
- 4 eggs
- 1 tsp. toasted sesame seeds
- 5 oz fresh shiitake mushroom caps, sliced
- 1 tbsp. apple cider vinegar
- 2 cups butternut squash, diced

- 2 cups fresh baby spinach leaves
- Cooking spray
- 4 ounces snow peas, ends trimmed
- Salt, to taste
- 1 (20-oz) bag frozen sweet potato fries
- 1 tsp. toasted sesame oil

Directions:

1. Whisk cider, gochujang, vinegar, maple syrup, cinnamon, and sesame oil in a bowl to prepare the chile sauce.
2. For the casserole, set the Ninja Foodi to Sear/Sauté mode on High heat.
3. Add oil to the foodi and heat it for 4 minutes.
4. Crack eggs in the pot without breaking the yolks and drizzle sesame seeds on top, then cook for 2 minutes.
5. Put on the Crisping Lid, then select Broil mode, set the cooking time to 1 minute. Hit the START/STOP button to initiate cooking.
6. Once done, slide the eggs into a sheet pan.
7. Switch the Ninja Foodi to the Sear/Sauté mode on High heat.
8. Add mushrooms and sauté for 4 minutes.
9. Stir in vinegar and cook for 1 minute, then transfer the mushrooms to the eggs.
10. Add remaining oil and butternut squash to the pot and sauté for 3 minutes.
11. Stir in spinach and snow peas, then put on the Crisping Lid.
12. Select Air Crisp mode, set the temperature to 390°F and cooking time to 6 minutes. Hit the START/STOP button to initiate cooking.
13. Transfer this mixture to the eggs and mushrooms, then empty the pot.
14. Place a Crisping Basket in the pot, add sweet potato fries, and grease them with cooking spray.
15. Cover the Crisping Lid and select Air Crisp mode, set the temperature to 390°F, and cooking time to 20 minutes. Hit the START/STOP button to initiate cooking.
16. Toss the sweet potato fries with salt and transfer to the veggies. Pour the chili sauce on top.
17. Serve.

CARAMELIZED BACON

COOKING TIME: 22 MIN | SERVES 6

INGREDIENTS:

- 1-pound bacon slices
- 1 cup light brown sugar, packed
- 1 tsp. black pepper

Directions:

1. Add bacon along with 1 cup water to the Ninja Foodi's cooking pot.
2. Put on the Pressure Lid and turn its Pressure handle to SEAL position.
3. Select Pressure Cook mode, set the pressure to High and cooking time to 2 minutes. Hit the START/STOP button to initiate cooking.
4. Once it's done, release the pressure quickly, then remove the lid.
5. Add black pepper and brown sugar, then cover with the Crisping Lid.
6. Select Air Crisp mode, set the temperature to 390°F and cooking time to 20 minutes. Hit the START/STOP button to initiate cooking.
7. Once done, remove the Crisping lid and transfer the bacon to a wire rack.
8. Allow the crispy bacon slices to cool for 10 minutes, then serve.

SHRIMP CASSEROLE

COOKING TIME: 14 MIN | SERVES 4

INGREDIENTS:

- 3 tbsp. butter, unsalted
- 1 cup Quick 5-Minute Grits
- 2 garlic cloves, minced
- 1 tsp. salt
- Black pepper, to taste
- 2 cups whole milk
- ½ cup cheddar cheese, shredded
- 2 tbsp. pickled jalapeño, minced
- 12 ounces frozen shrimp, peeled and deveined
- Cooking spray
- Chopped fresh chives (to garnish)

DIRECTIONS:

1. Preheat the Ninja Foodi at Sear/Sauté mode on High.
2. Add butter to melt for 4 minutes, then add garlic, grits, black pepper, and 1 tsp. salt.
3. Sauté for 3 minutes, then pour in 2 cups of water.
4. Put on the Pressure Lid and turn the pressure handle to the SEAL position.
5. Select Pressure Cook mode, set the pressure to High, and cooking time to 0 minutes. Hit the START/STOP button to initiate cooking.
6. Once it's done, release the pressure quickly, then remove the lid.
7. Add jalapeno, cheese, and milk, then mix well.
8. Transfer the grits to a bowl and empty the Ninja Foodi's pot.
9. Set the reversible rack inside the pot in the high position.
10. Toss shrimp with black pepper, salt, and cooking spray in a bowl.
11. Transfer the shrimp to the rack and put on the Crisping Lid.
12. Select Broil mode, set the cooking time to 10 minutes. Hit the START/STOP button to initiate cooking.
13. Toss the shrimp after every 5 minutes.
14. Divide the grits into 4 serving bowls.
15. Top the grits with shrimp and garnish with chives.
16. Serve warm.

CINNAMON BREAD STICKS

COOKING TIME: 25 MIN | SERVES 6

INGREDIENTS:

- 3 (8-inch) sub rolls, cut into eight pieces
- ½ cup heavy cream
- ½ cup whole milk
- 3 eggs
- 2 tbsp. sugar
- ½ tsp. salt
- 2 tbsp. unsalted butter, melted
- 1 tsp. cinnamon (ground)
- Cooking spray
- Warm maple syrup (to garnish)

DIRECTIONS:

1. Add 12 pieces of bread to the crisper basket at a time and place this basket in the Ninja Foodi's inner pot.
2. Put on the Crisping Lid and select Bake/Roast mode, set the temperature to 325°F, and cooking time to 7 minutes. Hit the START/STOP button to initiate cooking.
3. Remove the lid and transfer the slice to a plate, then continue roasting the remaining bread slices in the same manner.
4. Mix cream, milk, sugar, salt, melted butter, and eggs in a bowl.
5. Dip the breadsticks in the milk mixture and add 8 pieces to the crisping basket.
6. Place the basket in the Ninja Foodi's pot and put on the Crisping Lid.
7. Select Air Crisp mode, set the temperature to 390°F and cooking time to 9 minutes. Hit the START/STOP button to initiate cooking.
8. Once these pieces are done, continue cooking the remaining breadsticks in the same manner.
9. Garnish with maple syrup.
10. Serve.

SWEET ALMOND GRANOLA

COOKING TIME: 24 MIN | SERVES 12

INGREDIENTS:

- ½ cup peanut oil
- ½ cup agave syrup, light
- ½ cup brown sugar, light
- 1 tsp. salt
- 4 cups old-fashioned rolled oats
- 2 cups almonds, sliced
- ¾ cup dried sweet cherries
- Zest of 1 lime

Directions:

1. Mix salt, brown sugar, agave syrup, and peanut oil in the Ninja Foodi's inner pot.
2. Cook this mixture on Sear/Sauté on Medium heat for 4 minutes.
3. Stir in almonds and oats, then put on the Crisping Lid.
4. Select Air Crisp mode, set the temperature to 300°F and cooking time to 20 minutes. Hit the START/STOP button to initiate cooking.
5. Stir the granola after every 5 minutes.
6. Serve.

CHEESE POPPER EGG BAKE

COOKING TIME: 9 MIN | SERVES 4

INGREDIENTS:

- 4 eggs
- Cooking spray
- 1 (15-ounce) box frozen jalapeño poppers
- ¼ cup whole milk
- ½ tsp. salt
- 1 cup cheddar cheese, shredded

Directions:

1. Spread the poppers in the Crisping basket and set the basket in the Ninja Foodi's inner pot.
2. Spray the jalapeno poppers with cooking spray and cover with the Crisping Lid.
3. Put the Crisping Lid, select Air Crisp mode, set the temperature to 390°F, and cooking time to 3 minutes. Hit the START/STOP button to initiate cooking.
4. During this time, beat eggs with salt and milk in a bowl.
5. Once the poppers are cooked, remove the lid and pour the egg mixture over poppers.
6. Put the Crisping Lid, select Air Crisp mode, set the temperature to 390°F, and cooking time to 3 minutes. Hit the START/STOP button to initiate cooking.
7. Drizzle cheese over the eggs and continue Air Crisping for another 3 minutes.
8. Transfer the frittata to a plate.
9. Slice and serve warm.

HOMEMADE GREEK YOGURT

COOKING TIME: 12 HRS. 15 MIN | SERVES 16

INGREDIENTS:

- 8 cups whole milk
- ¼ cup plain yogurt starter

DIRECTIONS:

1. Mix ¼ milk with yogurt in a bowl and keep it aside.
2. Add remaining milk to the Ninja Foodi's inner pot.
3. Set the Ninja Foodi to Sear/Sauté Mode on Medium heat.
4. Warm up the milk for 15 minutes until its temperature reaches to 180°F.
5. Put on the Crisping Lid, then select dehydrate mode, set the temperature to 110°F, and cooking time to 12 hours. Hit the START/STOP button to initiate cooking.
6. After 20 minutes, add the reserved yogurt-milk mixture, then cover it with a plastic sheet.
7. Put on the Crisping Lid and then resume cooking.
8. Serve.

STICKY BREAKFAST CINNABUNS

COOKING TIME: 15 MIN | SERVES 10

INGREDIENTS:

DOUGH
- 2¼ tsp. instant yeast
- ½ cup water
- ½ cup whole milk
- 1 cup granulated sugar
- 1 cup unsalted butter, melted

- 1 large egg
- 1¼ tsp. salt
- 3½ cups all-purpose flour
- Cooking spray
- 2 tbsp. cinnamon, ground

ICING
- 1 cup confectioners' sugar
- 5 tbsp. heavy cream
- ½ tsp. salt

DIRECTIONS:

1. Mix yeast with water in a bowl and leave it for 5 minutes.
2. Beat egg, salt, half of the melted butter, ¼ cup granulated sugar, and milk in a bowl.
3. Stir in yeast mixture, and flour then mix well until it makes a dough.
4. Knead this dough on a working surface for 5 minutes.
5. Transfer this prepared dough to a greased bowl and cover with a plastic wrap.
6. Leave the dough in a warm place for 1 hour.
7. Knead the dough after 1 hour, then roll it into a 12x6 inches rectangle using a rolling pin.
8. Brush the top of the rolled 12x6 dough rectangle with the remaining butter.
9. Mix cinnamon with remaining sugar and drizzle this mixture on top.
10. Start rolling the sheet from the long side and slice this roll into 10 cinnamon rolls.
11. Place the cinnamon rolls on a plate, then cover them with a plastic sheet and leave for 30 minutes.
12. Transfer the cinnamon rolls to the reversible rack and place it in the Ninja Foodi's inner pot.
13. Put on the Crisping Lid, then select Bake/Roast mode, set the temperature to 375°F, and cooking time to 15 minutes. Hit the START/STOP button to initiate cooking.
14. Allow the cinnamon rolls to cool once cooked.
15. Meanwhile, mix the cream with sugar and salt in a small bowl.
16. Brush this icing over the baked cinnamon rolls.
17. Serve.

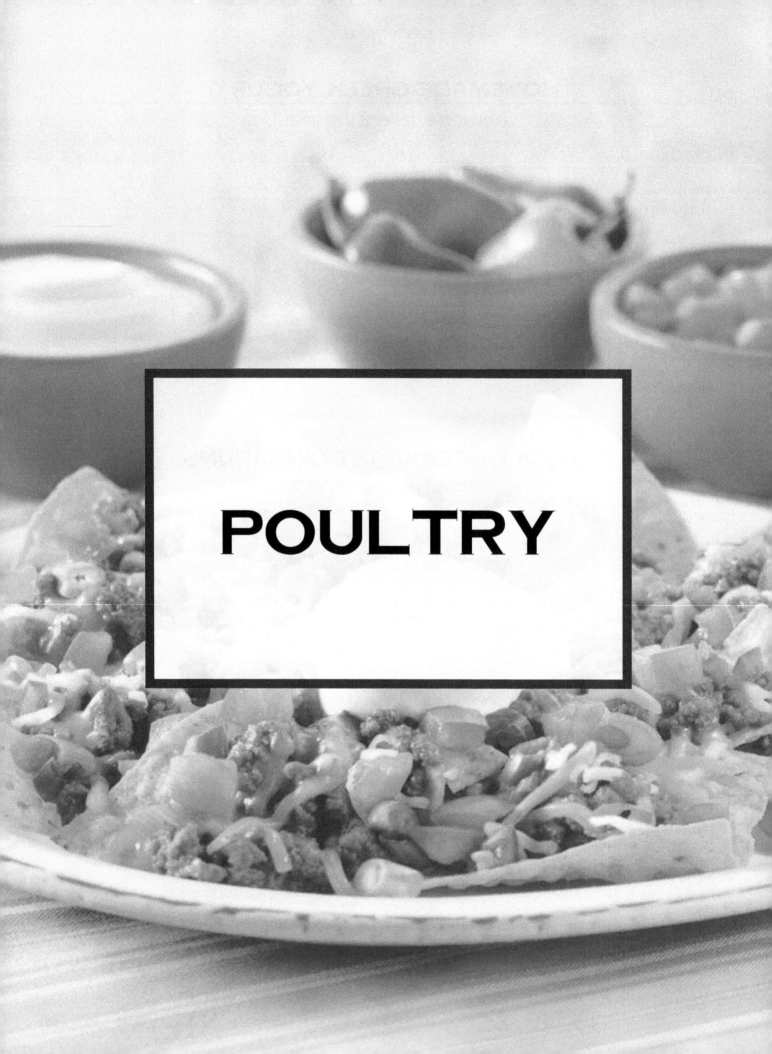

POULTRY

CHEESY CHICKEN NACHOS

COOKING TIME: 17 MIN | SERVES 4

INGREDIENTS:

- 4 skinless chicken breasts, frozen
- 1 (15 2/3 ounces) Jar red salsa
- 1 (15 ounces) can refried beans
- 1 tbsp. salt
- 2 tbsp. taco seasoning
- 4 ounces tortilla chips, divided
- 12 ounces cheddar cheese, grated
- Sour cream (to garnish)
- Guacamole (to garnish)
- Spring onions, sliced (to garnish)

Directions:

1. Add salsa and frozen chicken to the Ninja Foodi's cooking pot.
2. Put on the Pressure Lid and turn the pressure handle to the SEAL position.
3. Select Pressure Cook mode, set the pressure to High and cooking time to 12 minutes. Hit the START/STOP button to initiate cooking.
4. Once it's done, release the pressure quickly, then remove the lid.
5. Shred the cooked chicken with a fork, then add taco seasoning, salt, and refried beans.
6. Spread half of the tortilla chips on top of the chicken mixture and then drizzle half of the cheese on top.
7. Add another layer of the remaining tortilla chips and drizzle the cheese on top.
8. Put on the Crisping Lid, then select Air Crisp mode, set the temperature to 350°F, and cooking time to 5 minutes. Hit the START/STOP button to initiate cooking.
9. Once it's done, garnish with spring onions, sour cream, and guacamole.
10. Serve warm.

CREAMY CHICKEN PASTA

COOKING TIME: 8 MIN | SERVES 4

INGREDIENTS:

- 4 bacon slices
- 1-pound chicken breasts, boneless and skinless, diced
- 1 packet Ranch seasoning
- 16 ounces bowtie pasta
- 1 (32 ounces) carton chicken broth
- 4 ounces cream cheese
- 2 cups white cheddar cheese, shredded
- Fresh parsley (to garnish)

DIRECTIONS:

1. Add bacon to the Ninja Foodi's insert and sauté on Sear/Sauté mode on high heat until it is crispy.
2. Stir in chicken cubes and sauté until 5 minutes.
3. Add ranch seasoning, then toss well with the chicken.
4. Stir in pasta, and chicken broth, then put on the Pressure Lid.
5. Lock the lid and turn its pressure handle to the Seal Position.
6. Select Pressure cook mode, set the pressure to High and cooking time to 3 minutes. Hit the START/STOP button to initiate cooking.
7. Once it's done, release the pressure quickly, then remove the lid.
8. Stir in cheddar cheese and cream cheese.
9. Mix well and garnish with parsley.
10. Serve warm.

WHOLE ROAST CHICKEN WITH SAGE

COOKING TIME: 43 MIN | SERVES 4

INGREDIENTS:

- 4 pounds whole chicken, giblets removed
- 1 stick butter, cut into pieces
- Juice of 1 lemon, lemons reserved
- 5 fresh sage leaves
- 3 sprigs fresh thyme
- 2 sprigs fresh rosemary
- 2 garlic cloves, smashed
- 1 tbsp. ¼ tsp. salt
- ¼ tsp. black pepper
- 2 tbsp. instant flour

Directions:

1. Insert your fingers slowly under the chicken skin to create 2 pockets and add 4 pieces of butter to stuff the pockets.
2. Stuff the chicken with rosemary, thyme, sage, lemon halves, then fold the wings.
3. Place the stuffed chicken in the Ninja Foodi's Crisping Basket.
4. Set the basket inside and drizzle garlic, salt, and lemon juice on top.
5. Pour ½ water into the pot and put on the Pressure Lid.
6. Select Pressure Cook mode, set the pressure to High and cooking time to 23 minutes. Hit the START/STOP button to initiate cooking.
7. Once it's done, release the pressure quickly, then remove the lid.
8. Pour out the liquid to a bowl, empty the inner pot and return the chicken with the basket to the pot.
9. Brush the chicken with its own liquid, and drizzle black pepper and salt on top.
10. Now put on the Crisping Lid to cover the chicken.
11. Select Air Crisp mode, set the temperature to 390°F and cooking time to 17 minutes. Hit the START/STOP button to initiate cooking.
12. Once it is done, transfer the prepared chicken to a serving platter.
13. Switch the Ninja Foodi to the Sear/Sauté mode on Medium heat.
14. Pour in reserved cooking liquid and warm it up.
15. Mix instant flour with 2 tbsp. water in a bowl and pour it into the pot.
16. Cook this gravy for 3 minutes with occasional stirring. Pour gravy over the chicken.
17. Serve warm.

CHICKEN IN CREAMY PARMESAN SAUCE

COOKING TIME: 12 MIN | SERVES 4

INGREDIENTS:

- 1 tbsp. olive oil
- 2 pounds chicken breasts, cut into tenders
- 8 ounces white mushrooms, sliced
- ½ cup onion, diced
- 2 tbsp. butter, salted
- 2 tbsp. all-purpose flour
- 1 tbsp. garlic, minced
- 1 cup chicken broth
- ½ cup milk
- ½ tsp. salt
- ½ tsp. black pepper
- 4 cups spinach, cut into pieces
- 1 cup Parmesan cheese, grated

DIRECTIONS:

1. Add onions with olive oil to the Ninja Foodi's inner pot.
2. Switch it to Sear/Sauté mode on High heat and sauté the onions for 4 minutes.
3. Add chicken tenders, black pepper, and salt to the pot and cook it for 4 minutes.
4. Stir in mushrooms, garlic, and chicken broth and put on the Pressure Lid.
5. Select Pressure Cook mode, set the pressure to High and cooking time to 5 minutes. Hit the START/STOP button to initiate cooking.
6. When it's done, release the pressure quickly, then remove the lid.
7. Switch the Ninja Foodi to Sear/Sauté on High.
8. Mix milk and all-purpose flour in a bowl and pour it into the inner pot.
9. Stir in Parmesan cheese and butter, then cook for 2 minutes. Add spinach and cook until wilted.
10. Serve warm.

CITRUS GLAZED CHICKEN

COOKING TIME: 13 MIN | SERVES 4

INGREDIENTS:

- 4 skinless chicken breasts, boneless
- Zest and Juice from 2 lemons
- 1 tsp. salt
- 1 tsp. black pepper
- Cooking spray

Directions:

1. Add chicken breasts, lemon juice, black pepper, lemon zest, salt, and ½ cup water to the Ninja Foodi's inner pot.
2. Put on the Pressure Lid, and turn the pressure handle to the Seal position.
3. Select Pressure Cook mode, set the pressure to High and cooking time to 3 minutes. Hit the START/STOP button to initiate cooking.
4. Once it's done, release the pressure quickly, then remove the lid.
5. Empty the pot and place the chicken breasts in the reversible rack.
6. Place the rack in the inner pot and coat the chicken with cooking spray.
7. Put on the Crisping Lid, select Broil, and cook the chicken for 10 minutes.
8. Serve warm.

SAUCY THAI CHICKEN

COOKING TIME: 12 MIN | SERVES 4

INGREDIENTS:

- 4 chicken breasts, skinless
- 2 stalks of lemongrass, cut in half
- 2 garlic cloves, crushed
- 1 tbsp. ginger, grated
- 2 limes, juiced and zested
- Small bunch coriander, chopped

- 3 tbsp. soy sauce
- 2 tbsp. rice vinegar
- 2 tsp. fish sauce
- 1 red chili, finely chopped
- Salt and black pepper, to taste
- 1 cup jasmine rice, rinsed

- 1 1/3 cups (10 ½ ounces) chicken stock
- ½ tbsp. olive oil
- ½ tbsp. honey
- 1 cup broccoli florets
- Lime wedges (to garnish)

DIRECTIONS:

1. Mix lemongrass with ginger, garlic, lime zest, lime juice, rice vinegar, coriander stalk, 2 tbsp. soy sauce, fish sauce, rice vinegar, seasoning, and chili in a large bowl.
2. Place the chicken in this marinade, mix well and marinate for at least 30 minutes.
3. Add stock, 1 stalk of lemongrass from the marinade, and rice to the Ninja Foodi's inner pot.
4. Set a reversible rack in the pot and place the chicken breasts in the rack.
5. Put on the Pressure Lid and turn the pressure handle to the SEAL position.
6. Select Pressure Cook mode, set the pressure to High and cooking time to 2 minutes. Hit the START/STOP button to initiate cooking.
7. Release the pressure quickly when it is done, then remove the lid.
8. Add broccoli to the chicken and drizzle olive oil, 1 tbsp. soy sauce, and honey on top.
9. Place a Crisping Lid, then select Grill mode, set the cooking time to 10 minutes. Hit the START/STOP button to initiate cooking.
10. Transfer the rice, chicken, and broccoli to a plate.
11. Garnish with lemon wedges.
12. Serve warm.

HOT & CRISPY CHICKEN DRUMSTICKS

COOKING TIME: 20 MIN | SERVES 6

INGREDIENTS:

- 2 eggs, beaten
- ¼ cup hot sauce
- 3 cups self-rising flour
- 4 tsp. salt
- ½ tsp. black pepper

- 6 chicken drumsticks
- Cooking spray

Directions:

1. Preheat the Ninja Foodi on Air Crisp Mode at 390°F for 10 minutes.
2. Beat eggs with hot sauce in one bowl, and mix flour with black pepper and salt in another bowl.
3. First coat each drumstick with the flour, then dip them in the egg mixture and coat again with the flour mixture.
4. When all the drumsticks are coated, place them in the Crisping Basket.
5. Set the basket in the preheated Ninja Foodi and coat the drumsticks with cooking spray.
6. Put on the Crisping Lid and select Air Crisp mode, set the temperature to 390°F and cooking time to 20 minutes. Hit the START/STOP button to initiate cooking.
7. Serve warm.

CRUMBED CHICKEN CORDON BLEU

COOKING TIME: 15 MIN | SERVES 2

INGREDIENTS:

- 2 skinless chicken breasts, boneless
- 1 tsp. mayonnaise
- ½ tsp. Dijon mustard
- 4 deli ham, slices
- 4 Swiss cheese, slices
- 1 large egg

- 2 tsp. salt
- ½ cup breadcrumbs
- ¼ tsp. black pepper
- Cooking spray
- Chopped fresh parsley (to garnish)

DIRECTIONS:

1. Slice the chicken breast horizontally into half while keeping the two halves connected from one end.
2. Mix mustard and mayonnaise in a bowl.
3. Spread the chicken breasts into an open book and brush them with mayo mixture.
4. Add 2 ham slices on top of one half of each chicken breast and 2 slices of cheese on top of the bottom part of the chicken breast.
5. Start rolling each chicken breast from the narrow end towards the wider end.
6. Beat egg with a tsp. of salt in a bowl, and mix breadcrumbs with a tsp. of salt and black pepper in another bowl.
7. Dip the chicken roll in egg, then coat them with the breadcrumbs.
8. Place both the coated rolls with their seam side down in a Crisping Basket.
9. Transfer this basket to the Ninja Foodi's inner pot and spray the rolls with cooking spray.
10. Put on the Crisping Lid, select Air Crisp mode set the temperature to 390°F, and cooking time to 15 minutes. Hit the START/STOP button to initiate cooking.
11. Once done, garnish the rolls with parsley.
12. Enjoy.

PEPPER CHICKEN THIGHS

COOKING TIME: 25 MIN | SERVES 4

INGREDIENTS:

- 4 bone-in chicken thighs, skin-on
- Salt, to taste
- Black pepper, to taste
- Cooking spray

Directions:

1. Rub the chicken thighs with the black pepper and salt, then place them in the Crisping Basket.
2. Coat the skin on chicken thighs with the cooking spray, then transfer the basket to the Ninja Foodi's inner pot.
3. Put on the Crisping Lid, then select Air Crisp mode, set the temperature to 390°F, and cooking time to 25 minutes. Hit the START/STOP button to initiate cooking.
4. Once it's done, serve the chicken wings right away.

HONEY GLAZED ROASTED CHICKEN

COOKING TIME: 37 MIN | SERVES 4

INGREDIENTS:

- 1 (90oz) fresh uncooked chicken
- Juice of 2 lemons
- 2 ounces hot water
- 2 ounces honey
- 1 tbsp. 1 tsp. salt
- 1 tbsp. whole black peppercorns

- 5 sprigs fresh thyme
- 5 garlic cloves, peeled and smashed
- 1 tbsp. vegetable oil
- 2 tsp. black pepper

DIRECTIONS:

1. Tie the chicken legs with a cooking twin.
2. Mix lemon juice, honey, hot water, and 1 tbsp. salt in a bowl.
3. Pour this mixture into the Ninja Foodi's inner pot and add garlic thyme and whole peppercorns.
4. Set the chicken in the Crisping Basket and place this basket in the inner pot.
5. Put on the Pressure Lid and turn its pressure handle to the SEAL position.
6. Select Pressure Cook mode, set the pressure to High and cooking time to 22 minutes. Hit the START/STOP button to initiate cooking.
7. Once done, release the pressure naturally in 5 minutes, then do a quick release.
8. Brush the cooked chicken with vegetable oil, and rub it with black pepper and salt.
9. Put on the Crisping Lid, then select Air Crisp mode, set the temperature to 400°F, and cooking time to 15 minutes. Hit the START/STOP button to initiate cooking.
10. Serve warm.

TUSCAN CHICKEN FARFALLE

COOKING TIME: 9 MIN | SERVES 4

INGREDIENTS:

- 4 ¼ cups of chicken broth
- 1-pound skinless chicken breast, boneless and diced
- 12 ounces farfalle pasta
- 5 ounces fresh spinach
- 8 ounces cream cheese
- 1 cup parmesan cheese, shredded
- 1/2 cup sun dried tomatoes, chopped

- 1/4 cup fresh basil, chopped
- 1 tbsp. Italian seasoning
- 1 tbsp. garlic, minced
- 1 tsp. red pepper flakes
- 1/2 tsp. salt
- 1/2 tsp. black pepper

Directions:

1. Add garlic, black pepper, chicken broth, Italian seasoning, salt, sun-dried tomatoes, chicken, and pasta to the Ninja Foodi's inner pot.
2. Put on the Pressure Lid and turn the pressure handle to the SEAL position.
3. Select Pressure cook mode, set the pressure to the high and cooking time to 4 minutes. Hit the START/STOP button to initiate cooking.
4. Once the pasta is done, release the pressure in 5 minutes, then remove the lid.
5. Add red pepper flakes, cheese, cream cheese, and spinach.
6. Mix well and leave until spinach is wilted.
7. Garnish with basil.
8. Serve warm.

KATSU CURRY

COOKING TIME: 20 MIN | SERVES 4

INGREDIENTS:

- 16 ounces uncooked chicken breasts, pounded into cutlets
- Salt and black pepper, to taste
- 3 tbsp. flour
- 1 egg, whisked
- 2 2/3 ounces panko bread crumbs
- 3 tbsp. canola oil

- 7oz uncooked basmati rice, rinsed
- 12 2/3 ounces water
- 1 carrot, peeled, cut into cubes
- 1 small onion, peeled, cut into cubes
- 10 ½ ounces white potatoes, peeled, cut into cubes
- 14 ounces Katsu curry sauce

DIRECTIONS:

1. Preheat your Ninja Foodi at Sear/Sauté mode on High heat for 5 minutes.
2. Rub the chicken cutlets with black pepper and salt in a bowl.
3. Spread flour in a bowl, beat the egg in another and spread the crumbs in a third bowl.
4. Take one pounded chicken cutlet at a time and coat it with flour.
5. Dip the cutlet in the egg and then coat it with breadcrumbs. Repeat the same with the remaining cutlets.
6. Put a skillet with cooking oil on medium heat and sear the cutlets for 5 minutes per side.
7. Transfer the prepared cutlets to a plate lined with a paper towel.
8. Add rice and water to the Ninja Foodi's inner pot and place the reversible rack on top.
9. Spread the veggies in the rack for cooking.
10. Put on the Pressure Lid and turn the Pressure handle to the SEAL position.
11. Select Pressure Cook mode, set the pressure to High and cooking time to 10 minutes. Hit the START/STOP button to initiate cooking.
12. Once the rice is done, release the pressure quickly, then remove the lid.
13. Stir in veggies and curry sauce, then mix well. Add the chicken on top.
14. Serve warm.

SPICY CHICKEN TIKKA

COOKING TIME: 20 MIN + OVERNIGHT MARINADE | SERVES 6

INGREDIENTS:

MARINADE:
- 1 cup Greek yogurt
- 2 garlic cloves, smashed
- 1-inch ginger knob, peeled and grated
- 1 tsp. cumin (ground)
- 1 tsp. garam masala
- ½ tsp. turmeric (ground)
- ½ tsp. cayenne
- 1 tsp. salt
- 1½ lbs. boneless chicken thighs, cubed

SAUCE:
- 1 (14-oz.) can tomatoes, diced, with juice
- ½ yellow onion, diced
- 2 garlic cloves, smashed
- 1-inch ginger knob, peeled and grated
- 1 tsp. cumin (ground)
- 1 tsp. garam masala
- 1 tsp. sweet paprika
- 1 tsp. salt
- 1 tbsp. cornstarch

- ½ cup heavy cream

Directions:

1. Mix turmeric, garlic, ginger, yogurt, cayenne, garam masala, cumin, and salt in a large bowl. Stir in chicken cubes, then mix well to coat.
2. Cover the chicken cubes with a plastic wrap and refrigerate overnight.
3. Prepare the sauce the next day and add all its ingredients to the Ninja Foodi's insert.
4. Set the reversible rack inside and place the marinated chicken on the rack.
5. Put on the Pressure Lid and turn the pressure handle to the SEAL position.
6. Select Pressure Cook mode set the pressure to High and cooking time to 8 minutes. Hit the START/STOP button to initiate cooking.
7. Once it's done, release the pressure quickly, then remove the lid.
8. Put on the Crisping Lid and cook the chicken on BROIL mode for 10 minutes.
9. Transfer the chicken to a plate and switch the Ninja Foodi to SUATE/SEAR mode.
10. Mix cornstarch with water in a small glass bowl and pour into the sauce.
11. Cook and mix the sauce for 2 minutes or more until it thickens.
12. Pour the sauce over the chicken.
13. Serve warm.

CRISPY DUCK BREASTS

COOKING TIME: 15 MIN | SERVES 2

INGREDIENTS:

- 2 (1¼-lb.) duck breasts, with skin
- Salt, to taste
- Black pepper, to taste

DIRECTIONS:

1. Add Crisping Basket inside the Ninja Foodi and cover the Crisping Lid. Preheat it for 5 minutes on AIR CRISP mode at 400 °F.
2. Score the duck breasts and carve a crosshatch pattern on top of each.
3. Pat dry the duck and rub them with black pepper and salt.
4. Place the duck breasts in the Ninja Foodi, put on the Crisping Lid, and cook for 15 minutes in the preheated Ninja Foodi.
5. Serve warm.

CHICKEN SHRED SALSA & SPAGHETTI

COOKING TIME: 10 MIN | SERVES 4

INGREDIENTS:

- 1 (8-oz) pack spaghetti broken into 1" pieces
- 1 (28-oz) can chunky salsa
- 4 cups chicken stock
- 1 cup shredded chicken, pre-cooked
- ½ can black beans, rinsed
- Jalapeños (to garnish)
- Grated cheese (to garnish)
- Fresh cilantro, chopped (to garnish)

Directions:

1. Add salsa, stock, and spagetti to the Ninja Foodi's insert.
2. Put on the Pressure Lid and turn the pressure handle to the SEAL position.
3. Select Pressure Cook mode, set the pressure to High, and cooking time to 0 minutes. Hit the START/STOP button to initiate cooking.
4. Once it's done, release the pressure naturally for 10 minutes, then remove the lid.
5. Add the chicken and black beans into the pot and stir. Allow to sit for 2 more minutes.
6. Garnish with cheese, jalapenos and a sprinkle of cilantro.
7. Serve warm.

SPICY RAMEN WITH CHICKEN

COOKING TIME: 11 MIN | SERVES 2

INGREDIENTS:

- 3 tbsp. sunflower oil
- ½ yellow onion, diced
- 2 garlic cloves, smashed
- 3 dried red chiles
- 1 chipotle chile, minced
- 1 tsp. Shichimi togarashi
- ½ tsp. cayenne
- ½ tsp. chili powder
- ½ tsp. dry mustard
- ¼ tsp. smoked paprika
- 1 tbsp. Korean chile paste
- 1 large boneless chicken breast, cubed
- ½ tsp. chicken bouillon powder
- 1 (4-oz.) pack instant ramen noodles
- ½ tsp. salt
- 2 tsp. sugar
- 2 soft-boiled eggs, peeled and sliced
- Toasted sesame seeds(to garnish)
- Fresh cilantro, chopped (to garnish)

DIRECTIONS:

1. Heat oil in the Ninja Foodi's insert on SEAR/SAUTE mode on High.
2. Stir in garlic and onion, then sauté for 4 minutes.
3. Stir in chipotle, dried chiles, shichimi togarashi, paprika, dry mustard, chili powder, and cayenne.
4. Sauté for 1 minute, then mix well.
5. Whisk Korean chile paste with 1 cup water in a bowl.
6. Add chicken, bouillon powder, and Korean chile paste mixture.
7. Mix well and stir in noodles then cook for 4 minutes.
8. Put on the Crisping Lid to cover the noodles.
9. Select Air Crisp mode, set the temperature, and cooking time to 0 minutes. Hit the START/STOP button to initiate cooking.
10. Once it's done, release the pressure quickly, then remove the lid.
11. Add sugar and salt to the noodles, then mix well and transfer to a serving plate.
12. Add a rack to the Ninja Foodi and place the eggs in the rack then pour ½ cup water into the pot.
13. Put on the Pressure Lid and turn the pressure handle to the SEAL position.
14. Select Pressure Cook mode, set the pressure to High, and cooking time to 2 minutes. Hit the START/STOP button to initiate cooking.
15. Once it's done, release the pressure quickly, then remove the lid.
16. Drain and transfer the eggs to cold water and peel.
17. Serve the noodles with boiled eggs.
18. Serve warm.

HEARTY EGG NOODLES

COOKING TIME: 37 MIN | SERVES 4

INGREDIENTS:

- 14-oz. egg noodles
- ½ cup chicken stock
- ¼ cup oyster sauce
- 1 tbsp. soy sauce
- 2 tsp. cornstarch
- 1 tsp. toasted sesame oil
- ¼ cup vegetable oil
- 3 garlic cloves, smashed
- 1-inch ginger knob, peeled and grated
- 4 bok choy leaves, chopped
- 8 oz. fresh snow peas
- 2 medium carrots, shredded

Directions:

1. Add noodles to the crisper basket of the Ninja Foodi's insert.
2. Fill the Ninja Foodi's insert with water and switch the foodi to SEAR/SAUTE mode on High.
3. Cook the noodles for 30 minutes, then drain and rinse them under cold water.
4. Mix stock, sesame oil, cornstarch, soy sauce, and oyster sauce in a small bowl.
5. Empty the Ninja Foodi's insert and add oil, then switch the foodi to SEAR/SAUTE.
6. Add ginger, garlic, and bok choy to the oil and sauté for 1 minute.
7. Stir in snow peas and sauté for 2 minutes, then add carrots.
8. Cook for 1 and add noodles and cook for 1 minute.
9. Stir in oyster sauce mixture and cook for 3 minutes.
10. Serve warm.

CHILI CHICKEN WINGS

COOKING TIME: 10 MIN | SERVES 4

INGREDIENTS:

- ½ cup water
- ½ cup hot pepper sauce
- 2 tbsp. butter, unsalted, melted
- 1 ½ tbsp. apple cider vinegar
- 2 lbs. frozen chicken wings
- 1 oz. Ranch dressing mix
- ½ tsp. paprika
- Nonstick cooking spray

DIRECTIONS:

1. Add vinegar, hot sauce, and water to the Ninja Foodi's insert.
2. Place the chicken wings in the Ninja Foodi's Crisping Basket and set it in the Ninja Foodi.
3. Put on the Pressure Lid and turn the pressure handle to the SEAL position.
4. Select Pressure Cook mode, set the pressure to High, and cooking time to 5 minutes. Hit the START/STOP button to initiate cooking.
5. Once it's done, release the pressure quickly, then remove the lid.
6. Coat the wings with cooking spray, paprika, and dressing mix.
7. Put on the Crisping Lid to cover the chicken.
8. Select Air Crisp mode, set the temperature to 375 °F and cooking time to 5 minutes. Hit the START/STOP button to initiate cooking.
9. Once it's done, remove the lid.
10. Serve warm.

HOISIN CHICKEN ROLLS

COOKING TIME: 8 MIN | SERVES 4

INGREDIENTS:

- 1 ½ lb. ground chicken
- 1 cup of water
- ½ yellow onion, diced
- ¼ cup hoisin sauce
- ¼ cup of soy sauce
- 1 tsp. garlic, minced
- ¼ tsp. sesame oil
- ¼ tsp. ginger (ground)
- 5 oz. can water chestnuts
- 3 green onions, sliced
- 4 wraps, ready made

DIRECTIONS:

1. Fill the Ninja Foodi's insert with water and set the trivet inside then arrange the chicken on the trivet.
2. Put on the Pressure Lid and turn the pressure handle to the SEAL position.
3. Select Pressure Cook mode, set the pressure to High, and cooking time to 5 minutes. Hit the START/STOP button to initiate cooking.
4. Once it's done, release the pressure quickly, then remove the lid.
5. Empty the pot and return the chicken to the Ninja Foodi's insert.
6. Switch the Ninja Foodi to the SEAR/SAUTE MODE.
7. Stir in hoisin, onion, soy sauce, minced garlic, water chestnuts, ginger (ground), and sesame oil.
8. Sauté for 3 minutes, then add green onions.
9. Heat wraps and divide the mixture into equally into them. Roll up and serve warm.

PINEAPPLE CHICKEN WITH RICE

COOKING TIME: 30 MIN | SERVES 4

INGREDIENTS:

- 4 medium chicken thighs
- ¼ cup of water
- ½ cup honey
- 2 tbsp. ketchup
- ½ cup tamari
- 1 garlic clove, crushed
- ½ tsp. ginger
- 2 tbsp. cornstarch
- 8 oz. can pineapple chunks
- 3 cups cooked white rice

DIRECTIONS:

1. Add water, soy sauce, honey, ginger, ketchup and garlic to the Ninja Foodi's insert.
2. Place the trivet in the Ninja Foodi's insert and set the chicken on the trivet.
3. Brush the chicken with the pineapple juice.
4. Put on the Pressure Lid and turn the pressure handle to the SEAL position.
5. Select Pressure Cook mode, set the pressure to High, and cooking time to 25 minutes. Hit the START/STOP button to initiate cooking.
6. Once it's done, release the pressure quickly, then remove the lid.
7. Transfer the juicy chicken to a plate, then add pineapple and cornstarch to the cooking liquid.
8. Switch the Ninja Foodi to SEAR/SAUTE mode and cook for 5 minutes.
9. Stir in cooked white rice, and chicken then mix well.
10. Serve warm.

PESTO TOMATO CHICKEN

COOKING TIME: 25 MIN | SERVES 4

INGREDIENTS:

- 1 cup grape tomatoes, halved
- 4 chicken thighs, boneless
- 1 bunch asparagus, trimmed
- ½ cup chicken broth
- 6 oz. pesto sauce

Directions:

1. Add chicken, veggies, broth, and pesto to the Ninja Foodi's insert.
2. Put on the Pressure Lid and turn the pressure handle to the SEAL position.
3. Select Pressure Cook mode, set the pressure to High, and cooking time to 25 minutes. Hit the START/STOP button to initiate cooking.
4. Once it's done, release the pressure naturally, then remove the lid.
5. Serve warm.

QUICK & EASY ROAST CHICKEN

COOKING TIME: 60 MIN | SERVES 4

INGREDIENTS:

- 1 cup chicken broth
- 4 2/5 lb. chicken, frozen
- 1 onion, sliced
- 1 tsp. garlic salt
- 1 tsp. seasoned salt

Directions:

1. Add chicken broth and sliced onions to the Ninja Foodi's insert.
2. Set the trivet in the Ninja Foodi's insert and place the chicken on the trivet.
3. Put on the Pressure Lid and turn the pressure handle to the SEAL position.
4. Select Pressure Cook mode, set the pressure to High, and cooking time to 60 minutes. Hit the START/STOP button to initiate cooking.
5. Once it's done, release the pressure naturally, then remove the lid.
6. Drizzle the salt over the chicken and switch the Ninja Foodi to BROIL mode, and cook for 4 minutes.
7. Serve warm.

ITALIAN PARMESAN CHICKEN

COOKING TIME: 10 MIN | SERVES 4

INGREDIENTS:

- 2 boneless chicken breasts
- 2 cups Italian salad dressing
- 1/3 cup parmesan cheese, grated

Directions:

1. Add 1 cup Italian dressing and chicken breasts to the Ninja Foodi's insert.
2. Pour 1 cup of the Italian dressing and 1/3 parmesan cheese on top.
3. Put on the Pressure Lid and turn the pressure handle to the SEAL position.
4. Select Pressure Cook mode, set the pressure to High, and cooking time to 10 minutes. Hit the START/STOP button to initiate cooking.
5. Once it's done, release the pressure naturally, then remove the lid.
6. Serve warm.

TERIYAKI CHICKEN

COOKING TIME: 14 MIN | SERVES 2

INGREDIENTS:

- 1 cup chicken stock
- 1 cup long-grain white rice, rinsed
- ½ cup mixed veggies, frozen
- 1 tbsp. Adobo seasoning
- 1 head broccoli, cut into florets
- 2 8 oz. boneless chicken breasts
- 1 tbsp. olive oil
- ¼ cup teriyaki sauce
- 2 tsp. salt and black pepper

DIRECTIONS:

1. Add vegetables, Adobo seasoning, rice, chicken stock, black pepper, and salt to the Ninja Foodi's insert.
2. Place the reversible rack inside and set the chicken in it.
3. Put on the Pressure Lid and turn the pressure handle to the SEAL position.
4. Select Pressure Cook mode, set the pressure to High, and cooking time to 2 minutes. Hit the START/STOP button to initiate cooking.
5. Once it's done, release the pressure naturally for 10 minutes, then remove the lid.
6. Toss broccoli with black pepper, salt, and olive oil in a bowl.
7. Brush the chicken with teriyaki sauce and add broccoli around it.
8. Put on the CRISPING LID and cook on BROIL mode for 12 minutes.
9. Serve the chicken with rice.

EASY CHICKEN PARMIGIANA

COOKING TIME: 20 MIN | SERVES 3

INGREDIENTS:

- 2 eggs, whisked
- 3 chicken breasts, thawed
- ¼ cup parmesan cheese, grated
- ¼ cup bread crumbs
- ½ tsp. onion powder
- ½ tsp. Italian seasoning
- ½ tsp. garlic powder
- ½ cup mozzarella cheese, shredded
- ½ cup marinara sauce

DIRECTIONS:

1. Beat eggs in one bowl, mix breadcrumbs with Parmesan, onion and garlic powder in a bowl.
2. Dip the prepared chicken in egg and then coat with parmesan mixture.
3. Grease the Ninja Foodi's Crisping Basket with cooking spray and place the chicken inside.
4. Transfer the Ninja Foodi's Crisping Basket to the Ninja Foodi then put on the Crisping Lid.
5. Cook on AIR CRISP MODE for 18 minutes at 360 °F.
6. Once done, remove the lid and add marinara sauce and cheese on top.
7. Continue Air Crisping for 2 minutes, then garnish with Italian Seasonings.
8. Serve warm.

NINJA SHEPHERD'S PIE

COOKING TIME: 20 MIN | SERVES 4

INGREDIENTS:

- ½ onion, chopped
- 1 cup carrots, diced
- 1 1/3 cup chicken broth
- 1 cup celery, diced
- 3 tbsp. tomato paste
- 1 lb. lean ground turkey
- 2 cups cauliflower, chopped
- 2 tbsp. butter
- 2 cups red potatoes, peeled and chopped
- 1 tsp. Himalayan salt

Directions:

1. Grease the Ninja Foodi's insert with cooking spray and select the SEAR/SAUTE mode.
2. Stir in ground turkey and sauté for 5 minutes.
3. Add veggies and cook for 3 minutes.
4. Transfer the mixture to a round casserole dish.
5. Add 1/3 cup broth, ½ tsp salt, and tomatoes to the chicken and cover it with a foil sheet.
6. Add cauliflower, 1 cup broth, and potatoes to the Ninja Foodi's insert.
7. Place the trivet on top and set the casserole dish over it.
8. Put on the Pressure Lid and turn the pressure handle to the SEAL position.
9. Select Pressure Cook mode, set the pressure to High, and cooking time to 7 minutes. Hit the START/STOP button to initiate cooking.
10. Once it's done, release the pressure quickly, then remove the lid.
11. Remove the casserole dish and remove the potatoes and cauliflower to a bowl.
12. Mash the potatoes with a masher, then add ½tsp salt, 2 tbsp olive oil.
13. Add mashed potatoes on top of the turkey mixture.
14. Return the casserole to the trivet and put on the Crisping Lid.
15. Cook on BROIL mode for 5 minutes.
16. Serve warm.

BACON-WRAPPED CHICKEN BITES

COOKING TIME: 25 MIN | SERVES 4

INGREDIENTS:

- 1 lb. chicken tenderloins
- 1 package turkey bacon
- 2 oz. cheddar cheese, sliced
- 1 avocado, sliced
- Cooking oil spray
- Garlic powder, to taste
- Salt, to taste

DIRECTIONS:

1. Rub the chicken with salt and garlic powder.
2. Wrap each chicken piece with 2 bacon pieces and secure it with a toothpick.
3. Place the wrapped chicken in the Ninja Foodi's Crisping Basket and coat them with cooking spray.
4. Transfer the basket to the Ninja Foodi.
5. Put on the Crisping Lid and cook on AIR CRISP mode at 370 °F for 10 minutes.
6. Flip the chicken and continue cooking for 10 minutes.
7. Garnish with cheese on top.
8. Serve with avocado.

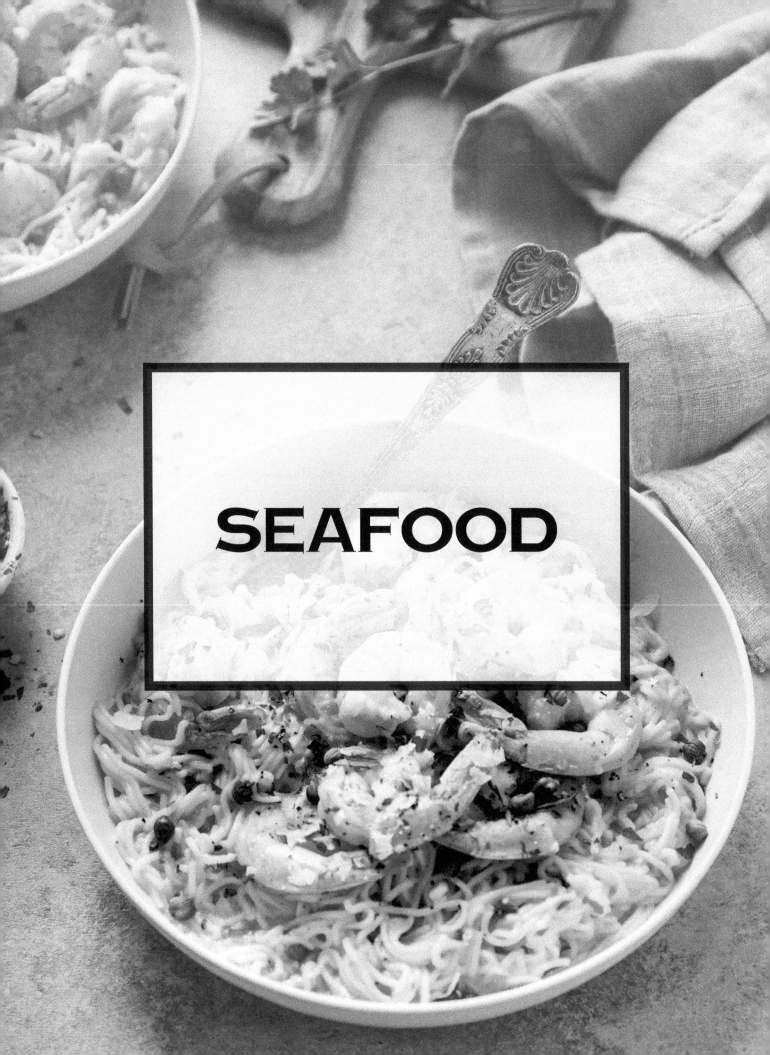

SEAFOOD

SHRIMP & SPAGHETTI SCAMPI

COOKING TIME: 7 MIN | SERVES 4

INGREDIENTS:

- 16 oz. frozen, shrimp, deveined
- 1 lb. spaghetti
- 1 cup dry white wine
- 1 lemon, juice, and zest
- 5 garlic cloves, chopped
- 3 cups water

- 1 stick butter
- 1 tsp. fresh parsley, chopped
- 1 tbsp. Parmesan grated
- Salt and black pepper, to taste
- 2 tbsp. olive oil

Directions:

1. Sauté shrimp with half of the butter in the Ninja Foodi's insert on SEAR/SAUTE mode for 2 minutes.
2. Stir in 1 cup wine, 3 cups water, salt, olive oil, and spaghetti.
3. Put on the Pressure Lid and turn the pressure handle to the SEAL position.
4. Select Pressure Cook mode, set the pressure to High, and cooking time to 5 minutes. Hit the START/STOP button to initiate cooking.
5. Once it's done, release the pressure quickly, then remove the lid.
6. Add remaining butter, shrimp, parsley, and lemon.
7. Leave it for 5 minutes, then garnish with Parmesan.
8. Serve warm.

THAI SHRIMP CURRY & RICE

COOKING TIME: 20 MIN | SERVES 4

INGREDIENTS:

- 2 tbsp. coconut oil
- 2 garlic cloves, smashed
- 1 green bell pepper, seeded, and sliced
- 1 orange bell pepper, seeded, and sliced
- 2 medium carrots, diced
- ½ yellow onion, diced
- 1 medium eggplant, peeled and diced

- ¼ cup green curry paste
- 1 (13.6-oz.) can coconut milk
- 2 tbsp. light brown sugar
- 2 tsp. salt
- 12 oz. frozen shrimp, peeled and deveined
- Cooking spray
- Steamed rice

DIRECTIONS:

1. Add oil to the Ninja Foodi's insert on SEAR/SAUTE mode.
2. Stir in garlic and sauté for 2 minutes.
3. Add bell peppers then sauté for 2 minutes.
4. Stir in onion and carrots then sauté for 2 minutes.
5. Add curry paste, and eggplant then cook for 2 minutes.
6. Pour in ¼ cup water and then put on the Pressure Lid and turn the pressure handle to the SEAL position.
7. Select Pressure Cook mode, set the pressure to High, and cooking time to 0 minutes. Hit the START/STOP button to initiate cooking.
8. Once it's done, release the pressure quickly, then remove the lid.
9. Switch the Ninja Foodi to the SEAR/SAUTE mode.
10. Stir in brown sugar, salt, and coconut milk, then cook for 2 minutes.
11. Transfer the eggplant curry to a bowl.
12. Set a reversible rack in the Ninja Foodi's insert and place the shrimp in it.
13. Coat the shrimp with salt and cooking spray, then put on the Crisping Lid.
14. Cook on AIR CRISP mode for 10 minutes at 390 °F.
15. Transfer the shrimp to the curry.
16. Serve warm with the rice.

SALT & PEPPER BROILED SALMON

COOKING TIME: 23 MIN | SERVES 2

INGREDIENTS:

- 1 lb. fresh asparagus, ends trimmed
- 2 tbsp. olive oil
- ½ tsp. salt
- Black pepper, to taste
- 1 (1-lb.) skin-on boneless salmon fillet,
- Cooking spray
- Lemon wedges (to garnish)

Directions:

1. Set the reversible rack in the Ninja Foodi's insert, put on the Crisping Lid, and preheat on BROIL mode for 5 minutes.
2. Toss with asparagus with ½ tsp salt and oil in a bowl.
3. Add asparagus to the reversible rack.
4. Rub the salmon with black pepper and salt, then place it in the rack.
5. Spray the salmon with cooking spray and put on the Crisping Lid.
6. Broil the salmon for 14 minutes on BROIL mode.
7. Flip the salmon and BROIL for another 4 minutes.
8. Serve warm with lemon wedges.

CRANBERRY SALMON RICE

COOKING TIME: 10 MIN | SERVES 4

INGREDIENTS:

- 1/3 cup dry cranberries
- 1/3 cup slivered almonds
- 1 ½ cups long-grain white rice, rinsed
- 1 ½ cups water
- Salt, to taste
- 4 (4-oz.) salmon fillets
- 1/3 cup panko bread crumbs
- 1 tbsp. honey
- 1/3 cup dry roasted sunflower seeds
- ¼ cup Dijon mustard
- 1 tbsp. parsley, minced

DIRECTIONS:

1. Mix mustard with sunflower seeds, honey, parsley, and breadcrumbs in a bowl.
2. Coat salmon fillet with the salt and wrap with the foil.
3. Add water, salt, rice, almond, and cranberries to the Ninja Foodi's insert, then set the reversible rack inside.
4. Place the foil packed salmon fillets in the rack.
5. Put on the Pressure Lid and turn the pressure handle to the SEAL position.
6. Select Pressure Cook mode, set the pressure to High, and cooking time to 2 minutes. Hit the START/STOP button to initiate cooking.
7. Once it's done, release the pressure naturally for 8 minutes, then remove the lid.
8. Coat the salmon with the breadcrumbs mixture and return to the rack.
9. Put on the Crisping Lid and cook on BROIL mode on High for 8 minutes.
10. Serve the salmon with rice.

GARLIC SHRIMP SKEWERS

COOKING TIME: 8 MIN | SERVES 2

INGREDIENTS:

- 1 lime, juiced
- 1 cup raw shrimp
- 1 garlic clove, minced
- 1/8 tsp. salt
- Black pepper, to taste
- 6 wooden skewers

DIRECTIONS:

1. Soak wooden skewers in a bowl for 20 minutes, then drain.
2. Preheat the Ninja Foodi on AIR CRISP mode at 350 °F for 5 minutes.
3. Add lime, garlic, shrimp, black pepper, and salt, then mix well.
4. Thread the cleaned shrimp on the skewers and place the skewers in the Ninja Foodi's Crisping Basket.
5. Transfer the basket to the Ninja Foodi and put on the Crisping Lid
6. Cook the shrimp skewers for 4 minutes on AIR CRISP mode and cook for another 4 minutes. Serve warm.

CREAMY MUSSELS

COOKING TIME: 25 MIN | SERVES 4

INGREDIENTS:

- 3 garlic cloves, smashed
- 1 cup cherry tomatoes, halved
- 2 tbsp. olive oil
- 2 shallots, sliced
- 2 cups heavy cream
- 1 ½ tsp. cayenne pepper
- 1 ½ tsp. black pepper
- 2 lbs. mussels, scrubbed and debearded
- 2 cups white wine
- 1 loaf sourdough bread, cut into slices

DIRECTIONS:

1. Add oil to the Ninja Foodi's insert and set the Ninja Food to SEAR/SAUTE mode on MD: HI.
2. Stir in garlic, cherry tomatoes, and shallots, then sauté for 5 minutes.
3. Add black pepper, cayenne, heavy cream, wine, and mussels, then mix well.
4. Put on the Pressure Lid and turn the pressure handle to the SEAL position.
5. Select STEAM mode, set the pressure to High, and the cooking time to 20 minutes. Hit the START/STOP button to initiate cooking.
6. Once it's done, release the pressure quickly, then remove the lid. Serve warm.

TUNA CAKES

COOKING TIME: 12 MIN | SERVES 4

INGREDIENTS:

- 2 packets (2.6 oz.) white tuna in water
- 1/4 cup breadcrumbs
- 1 oz. parmesan, shredded
- 1 oz. cheddar, shredded
- 1 large egg
- 2 tbsp. buffalo sauce
- 1 tsp. paprika
- 1/2 tsp. garlic powder
- 1/2 tsp. onion powder

DIRECTIONS:

1. Mix tuna with breadcrumbs, Parmesan, cheddar cheese, egg, buffalo sauce, paprika, garlic powder, and onion powder in a bowl.
2. Make four patties out of this tuna mixture.
3. Place the patties in the Ninja Foodi's Crisping Basket, spray them with cooking spray, and place the basket in the Ninja Foodi.
4. Put on the Crisping Lid and cook on AIR CRISP mode for 12 minutes at 400 °F.
5. Serve warm.

MISO RUBBED COD

COOKING TIME: 20 MIN | SERVES 4

INGREDIENTS:

- 4 (6 oz.) frozen cod fillets
- 1 cup yellow miso paste
- Cooking spray
- Sliced scallions (to garnish)
- Toasted sesame seeds (to garnish)
- Steamed rice (to serve)

Directions:

1. Rub the fish fillets with miso paste and place them on a plate.
2. Cover the fish with a plastic wrap and refrigerate for 8 hours.
3. Place the Crisping Basket in the Ninja Foodi, grease it with cooking spray.
4. Put on the Crisping Lid and preheat on BROIL mode for 5 minutes.
5. Place the cod in the Ninja Foodi's Crisping Basket, coat it with cooking spray, and put on the Crisping Lid.
6. Cook for 15 minutes on BROIL mode.
7. Garnish with sesame seeds and scallions.
8. Serve warm with steamed rice.

CAULIFLOWER SCALLOPS

COOKING TIME: 11 MIN | SERVES 2

INGREDIENTS:

- Cooking spray
- 1 lb. sea scallops
- 2 tbsp. butter, unsalted
- 1 cup chicken stock
- 2 tbsp. capers packed in brine, drained
- ¼ cup golden raisins
- 12 oz. fresh cauliflower florets
- 1 tbsp. instant flour

DIRECTIONS:

1. Grease the Ninja Foodi's insert with cooking spray and set the Ninja Foodi on SEAR/SAUTE mode.
2. Sear the scallops in the Ninja Foodi's insert for 3 minutes.
3. Add 1 tbsp butter and flip the scallops, then cook for 4 minutes and transfer to a plate.
4. Stir in ¾ cup stock and deglaze the pot. Stir in cauliflower, raisins, brine, and capers.
5. Put on the Pressure Lid and turn the pressure handle to the SEAL position.
6. Select Pressure Cook mode, set the pressure to High, and cooking time to 0 minutes. Hit the START/STOP button to initiate cooking.
7. Once it's done, release the pressure quickly, then remove the lid.
8. Add remaining 1 tbsp butter on top, then transfer the cauliflower to bowl.
9. Whisk remaining ¼ cup stock and flour in a bowl.
10. Pour this mixture into the Ninja Foodi's insert and switch the Ninja Foodi to SEAR/SAUTE mode.
11. Cook the mixture for 4 minutes until it thickens.
12. Serve the cauliflower and scallops with gravy.
13. Enjoy.

CRAWFISH ROTINI PASTA

COOKING TIME: 10 MIN | SERVES 6

INGREDIENTS:

- 1 (12-oz.) package rotini pasta
- 12 oz. crawfish tail meat, frozen
- 2 tbsp. Cajun seasoning
- 2 tsp. salt
- 2 tbsp. cornstarch
- 1 cup heavy cream
- ½ cup whole milk
- 1 cup Parmesan cheese, grated

Directions:

1. Add 5 cups water, salt, Cajun seasoning, crawfish meat, and pasta to the Ninja Foodi's insert.
2. Put on the Pressure Lid and turn the pressure handle to the SEAL position.
3. Select Pressure Cook mode, set the pressure to High, and cooking time to 0 minutes. Hit the START/STOP button to initiate cooking.
4. Once it's done, release the pressure naturally for 8 minutes, then remove the lid.
5. Mix milk with cream and cornstarch in a small bowl.
6. Pour this mixture into the pasta and drizzle cheese on top.
7. Put on the Crisping Lid and cook on AIR CRISP mode for 10 minutes at 390 °F.
8. Serve warm.

MISO GLAZED SALMON

COOKING TIME: 9 MIN | SERVES 4

INGREDIENTS:

- 1 cup jasmine rice, rinsed
- ¾ cup of water
- 4 frozen skinless salmon fillets
- 1 tsp. salt
- 2 tbsp. red miso paste
- 2 tbsp. butter softened
- 2 heads bok choy, cut in half
- ¼ cup mirin
- 1 tsp. sesame oil
- Sesame seeds (to garnish)

DIRECTIONS:

1. Add rice and water to the Ninja Foodi's insert and place the rack inside.
2. Rub the salmon with salt and place them on the rack.
3. Put on the Pressure Lid and turn the pressure handle to the SEAL position.
4. Select Pressure Cook mode, set the pressure to High, and cooking time to 2 minutes. Hit the START/STOP button to initiate cooking.
5. Once it's done, release the pressure quickly, then remove the lid.
6. Mix butter, mirin, bok choy, and sesame oil in a bowl.
7. Add this mixture on top of the fish and put on the Crisping Lid.
8. Cook on BROIL mode for 7 minutes.
9. Serve the salmon and bok choy with rice.

HONEY JALAPENO SALMON WITH RICE

COOKING TIME: 9 MIN | SERVES 4

INGREDIENTS:

- 1 small head broccoli, cut into florets
- 3 tbsp. olive oil
- 1 cup brown rice, rinsed
- ¾ cup water
- 4 (4-oz.) frozen skinless salmon fillets
- 1 tsp. black pepper (ground)
- 1 tsp. salt

- Juice of 2 limes
- 1 tsp. paprika
- 4 garlic cloves, smashed
- 2 jalapeño peppers, seeded and diced
- 2 tbsp. fresh parsley, chopped
- 2 tbsp. honey

Directions:

1. Add rice and water to the Ninja Foodi's insert and set the reversible rack on top.
2. Set the salmon fillets in the rack.
3. Put on the Pressure Lid and turn the pressure handle to the SEAL position.
4. Select Pressure Cook mode, set the pressure to High, and cooking time to 2 minutes. Hit the START/STOP button to initiate cooking.
5. Once it's done, release the pressure quickly, then remove the lid.
6. Transfer the salmon and rice to a plate, then keep them aside.
7. Toss broccoli with black pepper, salt, and 1 tbsp olive oil in a bowl.
8. Mix honey, 2 tbsp olive oil, lime juice, paprika, garlic, parsley, and jalapeno in a bowl.
9. Add cooked salmon to this honey sauce and rub it well.
10. Place the salmon and broccoli in the Ninja Foodi's insert.
11. Put on the pressure lid and cook on BROIL mode for 7 minutes.
12. Once done, release the pressure quickly, then remove the lid.
13. Serve the salmon with broccoli, rice, and parsley.

CRUMBED SHRIMP WITH A KICK

COOKING TIME: 7 MIN | SERVES 4

INGREDIENTS:

- 2 large eggs
- ¼ cup panko bread crumbs
- ¾ cup coconut flakes, unsweetened
- ½ cup all-purpose flour
- 2 tsp. ground black pepper

- ½ tsp. salt
- 24 shrimp, peeled and deveined
- 4 tbsp. Chili sauce

DIRECTIONS:

1. Mix flour with black pepper and salt in a bowl.
2. Beat eggs in one bowl and mix coconut flakes with breadcrumbs on a plate.
3. Coat the shrimp with flour, dip them in the egg and then coat with the breadcrumbs.
4. Place the shrimp in the Ninja Foodi's Crisping Basket and transfer it to the Ninja Foodi.
5. Put on the Crisping Lid and cook on AIR CRISP mode for 7 minutes at 400 °F.
6. Once it's done, remove the lid and transfer the shrimp to a plate.
7. Serve with chili sauce.

SPANISH MIXED PAELLA

COOKING TIME: 35 MIN | SERVES 4

INGREDIENTS:

- 1 (12 ounces) smoked sausage, sliced into rounds
- 1 medium yellow onion, diced
- 1 medium red bell pepper, seeded and diced
- 4 garlic cloves, minced
- 2 tsp. smoked paprika
- 3 (4 ounces) boneless, skinless chicken thighs, diced
- 2 cups short-grain white rice, rinsed
- 1½ cups chicken stock
- Pinch of saffron threads
- 1 cup frozen sweet peas
- 1 tsp. salt
- 8 ounces frozen tail-on shrimp, peeled and deveined
- Chopped fresh parsley (to garnish)
- Smoked paprika (to garnish)

Directions:

1. Add sausage to the Crisping Basket and place this basket in the Ninja Foodi's inner pot.
2. Put on the Crisping Lid, then select Air Crisp mode, set the temperature to 390°F, and cooking time to 10 minutes. Hit the START/STOP button to initiate cooking.
3. Remove the Crisping Basket from the inner pot and transfer the sausage to a plate.
4. Switch the Ninja Food to Sear/Sauté mode on High heat.
5. Add bell pepper and onion to the inner pot and sauté for 8 minutes.
6. Stir in paprika and garlic, then sauté for 4 minutes.
7. Add saffron, stock, and rice, then put on the Pressure Lid.
8. Turn the pressure handle to the SEAL position.
9. Select Pressure Cook mode, set the pressure to High and cooking time to 3 minutes. Hit the START/STOP button to initiate cooking.
10. Once it's done, then release the pressure quickly, then remove the lid.
11. Add peas, salt, shrimp, and sausage on top, then put on the Crisping Lid.
12. Select Air Crisp mode, set the temperature to 390°F and cooking time to 8 minutes. Hit the START/STOP button to initiate cooking.
13. Once the rice is done, remove the crisping lid.
14. Garnish with parsley and paprika.
15. Serve warm.

MARYLAND SPICED SHRIMP

COOKING TIME: 10 MIN | SERVES 4

INGREDIENTS:

- 1 tbsp. olive oil
- 2 tsp. Maryland-style seafood spice
- 1 (12-oz.) bag frozen tail-on shrimp
- Fresh lemon wedges (to garnish)

DIRECTIONS:

1. Place the reversible rack inside the Ninja Foodi's insert. Put on the Crisping Lid and preheat on BROIL mode for 5 minutes.
2. Toss tail-on shrimp with oil and spices in a bowl to coat.
3. Add the shrimp to the rack and put on the Crisping Lid.
4. Cook on BROIL mode for 10 minutes.
5. Flip the shrimp once cooked halfway through.
6. Serve warm with lemon wedges.

SNAPPER DINNER

COOKING TIME: 1 HR 32 MIN | SERVES 6

INGREDIENTS:

- ½ tbsp. dry mustard
- ¼ tbsp. ground nutmeg
- 6 tbsp. butter
- 3 tbsp. almond flour
- 1½ tsp. fresh lemon juice
- 1 cup cheddar cheese, shredded
- 1 tsp. salt
- 1¼ cups unsweetened almond milk
- 3 lbs. snapper fillets

Directions:

1. Add butter to Ninja Foodi's insert and preheat the Ninja Foodi on SEAR/SAUTE mode on MD: HI pressure.
2. Stir in salt, nutmeg, mustard, and flour, then mix well for 2 minutes.
3. Add milk, cheese, and lemon juice, then mix well until the cheese is melted.
4. Place fish in the sauce and baste it a little, then put on the lid.
5. Select Slow Cook mode, set the pressure to HI, and cooking time to 1 hour 30 minutes. Hit the START/STOP button to initiate cooking.
6. Once it's done, remove the lid.
7. Serve warm.

CREAMY SPINACH SCALLOPS

COOKING TIME: 10 MIN | SERVES 4

INGREDIENTS:

- ¾ cup heavy whipping cream
- 1 (10-oz.) pack spinach
- 12 sea scallops
- 1 tbsp. tomato paste
- 1 tsp. garlic, minced
- 1 tbsp. basil, chopped
- Salt and ground black pepper, to taste

DIRECTIONS:

1. Coat the scallops with salt, black pepper, and olive.
2. Toss spinach with butter in a baking pan and top it with scallops.
3. Whisk cream with black pepper, salt, basil, garlic, and tomato paste.
4. Spread this cream mixture over the scallops.
5. Place the reversible rack inside the Ninja Foodi's insert and set the pan over it.
6. Put on the Crisping Lid to cover the pot
7. Select Air CRIP mode, set the temperature to 350 °F and cooking time to 10 minutes. Hit the START/STOP button to initiate cooking.
8. Once it's done, remove the lid.
9. Serve warm.

CREAMY SEA BASS

COOKING TIME: 15 MIN | SERVES 4

INGREDIENTS:

- 1 red onion; chopped
- 1 tbsp. parsley; chopped
- 1 lb. sea bass fillets; boneless and cubed
- 1 cup coconut cream
- 1 tsp. olive oil
- Black pepper and salt to the taste

Directions:

1. Sauté onions with oil in the Ninja Foodi's insert on SEAR/SAUTE mode on MD: HI for 5 minutes.
2. Stir in seabass, coconut cream, black pepper and salt.
3. Put on the Pressure Lid and turn the pressure handle to the SEAL position.
4. Select Pressure Cook mode, set the pressure to High, and cooking time to 10 minutes. Hit the START/STOP button to initiate cooking.
5. Once it's done, release the pressure naturally, then remove the lid.
6. Garnish with parsley.
7. Serve warm.

SAUCY COD FILLETS

COOKING TIME: 15 MIN | SERVES 4

INGREDIENTS:

- 1 tbsp. chicken stock
- 1 tbsp. ginger, grated
- 2 tbsp. rice vinegar
- 2 tbsp. soy sauce
- Salt, to taste
- Black pepper, to taste
- 6 scallions, green parts, sliced
- 4 skinless cod fillets

DIRECTIONS:

1. Mix rice vinegar, ginger, chicken stock, and soy sauce in a bowl.
2. Rub the cod fillets with salt and black pepper.
3. Add oil to the Ninja Foodi's insert and heat it on SEAR/SAUTE mode on MD: HI for 5 minutes.
4. Stir in soy mixture and place the fillets in the Ninja Foodi's insert.
5. Put on the Pressure Lid and turn the pressure handle to the SEAL position.
6. Select Pressure Cook mode, set the pressure to LO, and cooking time to 10 minutes. Hit the START/STOP button to initiate cooking.
7. Once it's done, release the pressure naturally, then remove the lid.
8. Garnish with scallions.
9. Serve warm.

CLAMS NOODLES

COOKING TIME: 24 MIN | SERVES 4

INGREDIENTS:

- 4 bacon strips, cut into cubes
- 2 garlic cloves, smashed
- 2 shallots, minced
- 1-inch ginger knob, peeled and grated
- ¼ cup breadcrumbs
- ¼ cup Parmesan cheese, grated
- 2 cups chicken stock
- ¼ cup dry white wine
- 1 lb. scrubbed Manila clams
- 2 (4-oz.) packages instant ramen noodles
- Chopped parsley (to garnish)
- Red pepper flakes (to garnish)

Directions:

1. Sauté bacon in the Ninja Foodi's insert on SEAR/SAUTE mode on high for 4 minutes.
2. Stir in ginger, shallots, and garlic for 5 minutes.
3. Transfer half of the bacon mixture to a bowl and add Parmesan and breadcrumbs, then mix well.
4. Add wine and stock, then deglaze the pot, then add clams.
5. Put on the Pressure Lid and turn the pressure handle to the SEAL position.
6. Select Pressure Cook mode, set the pressure to High, and cooking time to 6 minutes. Hit the START/STOP button to initiate cooking.
7. Once it's done, release the pressure naturally, then remove the lid.
8. Push the cooked clams to one side and add noodles to the Ninja Foodi's insert.
9. Switch the Ninja Foodi to SEAR/SAUTE mode on High then sauté for 4 minutes.
10. Spread the breadcrumb mixture on top and cover the Crisping Lid.
11. Cook on BROIL mode for 5 minutes until golden brown.
12. Garnish with parsley, red pepper flakes, and basil.
13. Serve warm.

CREAMY COCONUT TROUT

COOKING TIME: 15 MIN | SERVES 4

INGREDIENTS:

- 2 tbsp. parsley, chopped
- 2 tsp. olive oil
- 2 tsp. garlic, minced
- 4 trout fillets, skinless and boneless
- 1/2 cup coconut milk
- Black pepper and salt to taste

DIRECTIONS:

1. Grease a suitable baking pan with cooking spray and add coconut milk, black pepper, salt, garlic, olive oil, and parsley.
2. Place the cleaned trout fillet in the baking pan and keep it aside.
3. Add water to the Ninja Foodi's insert and set the reversible rack inside.
4. Put on the Pressure Lid and turn the pressure handle to the SEAL position.
5. Select BAKE/ROAST mode, set the temperature to 380 °F, and cooking time to 15 minutes. Hit the START/STOP button to initiate cooking.
6. Once it's done, release the pressure naturally, then remove the lid.
7. Serve warm.

SHRIMP RED CURRY

COOKING TIME: 18 MIN | SERVES 4

INGREDIENTS:

- 1 tbsp. olive oil
- 1 bunch scallions, sliced
- ¼ cup red curry paste
- 2 tbsp. water
- 1 cup peas
- 1 red bell pepper, diced
- 1 lb. shrimp, peeled and deveined
- 1 (14-oz.) can full-fat coconut milk
- Salt, to taste

DIRECTIONS:

1. Mix the red curry paste with water in a mixing bowl.
2. Add oil to the Ninja Foodi's insert and heat on SEAR/SAUTE mode on MD: HI pressure for 5 minutes.
3. Stir in scallions, then sauté for 3 minutes.
4. Add bell pepper, peas, shrimp, and curry paste.
5. Mix well and sauté for 5 minutes.
6. Add coconut milk and salt, and cook for 5 minutes.
7. Serve warm.

SALMON FISH PIE

COOKING TIME: 42 MIN | SERVES 4

INGREDIENTS:

- 2 lbs. potatoes, peeled and cut into chunks
- 8 2/3 oz. water
- 1 2/3 oz. butter
- 2 ½ fl. oz. milk
- 1/2 tsp. salt
- Black pepper, to taste
- 1 2/3 oz. butter
- 1 medium onion, peeled and chopped
- 1 2/3 oz. plain flour
- 5 ¼ oz. white wine
- 12 ¼ oz. milk
- 5 ¼ oz. single cream
- 5 ¼ oz. broccoli, cut into l florets
- 17 ½ oz. skinless salmon, cut into cubes
- 7oz. peeled prawns, cooked
- 2 tbsp. fresh parsley
- 1 2/3 oz. grated Gruyere cheese

DIRECTIONS:

1. Add potatoes and water to the Ninja Foodi's insert
2. Put on the Pressure Lid and turn the pressure handle to the SEAL position.
3. Select Pressure Cook mode, set the pressure to High, and cooking time to 7 minutes. Hit the START/STOP button to initiate cooking.
4. Once it's done, release the pressure naturally, then remove the lid.
5. Drain the boiled potatoes and add them to a bowl.
6. Mash the potatoes with a potato masher, then add black pepper, salt, milk, and butter.
7. Then mix well and keep it aside.
8. Empty the Ninja Foodi and switch it to SEAR/SAUTE mode.
9. Add onion and butter to the Ninja Foodi's insert and sauté for 7 minutes.
10. Stir in flour and sauté for 1 minute.
11. Add cream, milk, and wine, then mix well and cook until the sauce thickens.
12. Stir in broccoli and cook for 2 minutes.
13. Add prawns, salmon, and parsley to the Ninja Foodi's insert.
14. Mix well and cook for 5 minutes, then spread the mashed potatoes and grated cheese on top.
15. Put on the Crisping Lid and cook on BAKE/ROAST mode for 20 minutes.
16. Serve warm.

GINGER SALMON

COOKING TIME: 30 MIN | SERVES 4

INGREDIENTS:

- 3 green chilies, chopped
- 1 lb. salmon fillets
- 2 tbsp. ginger-garlic paste
- Ground black pepper and salt to taste
- ¾ cup butter, melted

Directions:

1. Rub the salmon with ginger paste, black pepper, and salt.
2. Grease a suitable pan with cooking spray and place the salmon in the pan.
3. Drizzle chilies and butter over the salmon.
4. Add water to the Ninja Foodi's insert and set the reversible rack inside.
5. Put on the Pressure Lid and turn the pressure handle to the SEAL position.
6. Select BAKE/ROAST mode, set the temperature to 360 °F, and cooking time to 30 minutes. Hit the START/STOP button to initiate cooking.
7. Once it's done, release the pressure naturally, then remove the lid.
8. Serve warm.

SHRIMPY RICE NOODLES

COOKING TIME: 34 MIN | SERVES 6

INGREDIENTS:

- 1 (14-oz.) package rice stick noodles
- ¼ cup olive oil
- ½ cup of fish sauce
- 1/3 cup tamarind paste
- Juice of 1 lime
- 1/3 cup of sugar
- 2 tbsp. rice vinegar
- 12 frozen raw shrimp, peeled and deveined
- 3 garlic cloves, smashed
- 2 large whole dried shrimp, finely chopped
- ½ cup carrots, shredded
- 6 leaves bok choy, julienned
- 2 large eggs, beaten
- Cooking spray
- ½ cup salted peanuts, chopped
- Chopped fresh cilantro (to garnish)
- Lime wedges (to garnish)

DIRECTIONS:

1. Add noodles and enough water to cover the noodles to Ninja Foodi's insert.
2. Cook the noodles on SEAR/SAUTE mode on High for 20 minutes or more until soft.
3. Drain the noodles, then toss them with oil in a bowl.
4. Empty the inner pot and add oil to heat on SEAR/SAUTE mode.
5. Stir in garlic and dried shrimp, then sauté for 1 minute.
6. Add carrots, then sauté for 2 minutes and add bok choy leaves.
7. Cook for 4 minutes, then stir in eggs and cook for 1 minute.
8. Stir well, then add noodles to the pot and cook for 3 minutes.
9. Set the reversible rack in the Ninja Foodi's insert in a high position and set the shrimp over it.
10. Pour the marinade over the shrimp and put on the Crisping Lid.
11. Cook on AIR CRISP mode for 7 minutes at 390 °F.
12. Remove the crisping lid and cook for 1 minute and garnish with cilantro and lime wedges.
13. Serve warm.

BEEF, LAMB & PORK

BEEF MOSTACCIOLI BAKE

COOKING TIME: 13 MIN | SERVES 6

INGREDIENTS:

- 1 tsp. olive oil
- 1/2 cup onions, diced
- 1 lb. lean ground beef
- 1 tbsp. garlic- minced
- 1 tsp. sugar
- 1 tbsp. Italian seasoning
- 1/2 tsp. red pepper flakes

- 29 oz. beef broth
- 1 cup of water
- 1 (24 oz.) jar of pasta sauce
- 1 lb. dried mostaccioli noodles
- 2 cups mozzarella cheese, shredded

DIRECTIONS:

1. Add oil to the Ninja Foodi's insert and preheat it on SEAR/SAUTE mode on HI.
2. Stir in garlic, beef, and onions, then sauté until brown.
3. Add pasta sauce, red pepper flakes, pasta, beef broth, 1 cup water, sugar, and Italian seasoning.
4. Put on the Pressure Lid and turn the pressure handle to the SEAL position.
5. Select Pressure Cook mode, set the pressure to High, and cooking time to 3 minutes. Hit the START/STOP button to initiate cooking.
6. Once it's done, release the pressure naturally, then remove the lid.
7. Mix well and add 1 cup mozzarella cheese on top, then switch the Ninja Foodi to the BROIL mode.
8. Put on the Crisping Lid and cook for 5 minutes until melted.
9. Serve warm.

BEEF PICADILLO

COOKING TIME: 23 MIN | SERVES 4

INGREDIENTS:

- 2 lbs. ground beef
- 2 tbsp. olive oil
- 1 yellow onion, diced
- 1 green bell pepper, diced
- 4 cloves garlic, minced
- 1 cup beef broth
- 8 oz. can tomato sauce

- 6 oz. can tomato paste
- 1/4 cup white wine vinegar
- 10 jalapeño stuffed olives, chopped
- 2 oz. raisins
- 1/2 tbsp. cumin
- 1 tsp. dried oregano
- Salt and black pepper, to taste

DIRECTIONS:

1. Add olive oil to the Ninja Foodi's insert and preheat in on SEAR/SAUTE mode.
2. Stir in bell pepper, and onion then sauté for 8 minutes.
3. Add garlic, then sauté for 1 minute.
4. Stir in ground beef, then sauté until it turns brown.
5. Put on the Pressure Lid and turn the pressure handle to the SEAL position.
6. Select Pressure Cook mode, set the pressure to High, and cooking time to 8 minutes. Hit the START/STOP button to initiate cooking.
7. Once it's done, release the pressure quickly, then remove the lid.
8. Garnish with cilantro.
9. Serve warm.

GARLICKY LAMB RACK

COOKING TIME: 15 MIN | SERVES 4

INGREDIENTS:

- 18 oz. hand cut rack of lamb
- 1 large onion
- 4 tbsp. garlic paste
- 3 garlic cloves
- 2-star anise
- 3 ½ oz. water

- 1 tbsp. chili powder
- ½ tbsp. turmeric powder
- 1 tbsp. garam masala
- 1 tbsp. ginger paste
- 1 tbsp. garlic paste
- 1 tbsp. sunflower oil

DIRECTIONS:

1. Finely chop the onion in the food processor
2. Transfer the onion to the Ninja Foodi's insert and add water, lamb, star anise, cloves, and garlic paste.
3. Put on the Pressure Lid and turn the pressure handle to the SEAL position.
4. Select Pressure Cook mode, set the pressure to High, and cooking time to 5 minutes. Hit the START/STOP button to initiate cooking.
5. Once it's done, release the pressure naturally, then remove the lid.
6. Transfer the cooked lamb to a plate using a slotted spoon.
7. Mix turmeric powder, chili powder, ginger, and garlic paste, and garam masala in a bowl.
8. Rub this mixture on the lamb racks.
9. Set the reversible rack in the Ninja Foodi's insert and place the lamb in the rack.
10. Drizzle a tbsp oil over the lamb and put on the Crisping Lid.
11. Cook on AIR CRISP mode for 395 °F for 10 minutes.
12. Serve warm.

ROASTED BEEF WITH POTATOES

COOKING TIME: 60 MIN | SERVES 4

INGREDIENTS:

Beef:
- 2.2 lbs. beef roast
- 1 tbsp. olive oil
- Salt, to taste
- Black pepper, to taste

Potatoes:
- 15 small Charlotte potatoes
- 2 tbsp. olive oil
- Salt, to taste
- Black pepper, to taste
- 6 whole garlic cloves

DIRECTIONS:

1. Slice the potatoes in half and rub them with oil, garlic cloves, salt, and black pepper.
2. Place the potatoes in the Ninja Foodi's insert and set the reversible rack on top.
3. Set the beef on the rack and put on the Crisping Lid.
4. Select BAKE/ROAST mode, set the temperature to 428 °F, and cooking time to 30 minutes. Hit the START/STOP button to initiate cooking.
5. Reduce the temperature to 392 °F and cook for 30 minutes.
6. Once done, remove the lid and serve warm.

MEATBALL PASTA CASSEROLE

COOKING TIME: 22 MIN | SERVES 10

INGREDIENTS:

- 23 oz. beef mince
- 2 eggs
- ¼ cup parmesan cheese, grated
- ¼ cup milk
- ⅓ cup seasoned bread crumbs
- 1 tbsp. fresh parsley, chopped
- 2 tsp. granulated garlic
- 2 tsp. salt
- 3 tbsp. olive oil
- 5 ⅛ cup (47 ½ oz) marinara sauce
- 1 ½ cup water
- 1 ½ cup dry red wine
- 2 cups dry cavatappi pasta
- 1 ½ cup ricotta cheese
- ½ cup mozzarella, grated

DIRECTIONS:

1. Mix beef mince with eggs, milk, Parmesan cheese, breadcrumbs, salt, garlic, and parsley in a bowl.
2. Make 20 meatballs out of this beef mixture and keep them aside.
3. Add oil to the Ninja Foodi's insert and preheat it for 5 minutes on SEAR/SAUTE mode.
4. Stir in meatballs and sear them until golden brown.
5. Add pasta, water, wine, and marinara sauce.
6. Put on the Pressure Lid and turn the pressure handle to the SEAL position.
7. Select Pressure Cook mode, set the pressure to LOW, and cooking time to 2 minutes. Hit the START/STOP button to initiate cooking.
8. Once it's done, release the pressure naturally, then remove the lid.
9. Switch the Ninja Foodi to SEAR/SAUTE mode and cook for 10 minutes.
10. Drizzle mozzarella and ricotta cheese on top.
11. Put on the Pressure Lid and turn the pressure handle to the SEAL position.
12. Select BAKE/ROAST mode, set the temperature to 320 °F, and cooking time to 5 minutes. Hit the START/STOP button to initiate cooking.
13. Once it's done, release the pressure naturally, then remove the lid.
14. Serve warm.

MUSTARD RUBBED PORK TENDERLOIN

COOKING TIME: 20 MIN | SERVES 4

INGREDIENTS:

- 1 large egg, beaten
- ½ cup mayonnaise
- ¼ cup grainy mustard
- ½ tsp. black pepper
- ½ cup all-purpose flour
- 1 tsp. salt
- 2 (1-lb.) pork tenderloins, cut into thirds
- Cooking spray

DIRECTIONS:

1. Beat egg with mustard, mayonnaise, and black in a bowl.
2. Mix flour with salt in another shallow bowl.
3. Set a Crisping Basket in the Ninja Foodi's insert and put on the Crisping Lid.
4. Preheat the Ninja food on Broil mode for 5 minutes.
5. Dredge the tenderloin chunks through the flour mixture then coat them with mayonnaise mixture.
6. Place the coated tenderloin chunks in the Crisping Basket.
7. Cover with the Crisping Lid and cook on BAKE/ROAST mode for 15 minutes at 375 °F.
8. Remove the tenderloins from the foodi and slice them crosswise.
9. Serve warm.

LAMB CHOPS WITH SAFFRON RICE

COOKING TIME: 12 MIN | SERVES 2

INGREDIENTS:

- 4 lamb chops
- 2 tbsp. olive oil
- 2 garlic cloves, crushed
- 1 tsp. zaatar
- 1/2 tsp. Urfa chili
- 1 lemon, zest, and juice
- Salt and black pepper, to taste

- 8 2/3 oz. basmati rice, rinsed
- 10 ½ oz. chicken stock
- 2 green cardamom pods
- 1 pinch saffron
- 1 cinnamon stick
- 1 bay leaf
- 2 zucchinis, sliced diagonally

- 1 tbsp. olive oil

DIRECTIONS:

1. Mix garlic with lemon zest, juice, olive oil, chili, zaatar, and seasoning in a bowl.
2. Place lamb chops in the bowl and rub the seasoning well. Cover chops and marinate for 1 hour.
3. Add rice, stock, saffron, cardamom, bay leaf, and cinnamon stick to the Ninja Foodi's insert.
4. Set the reversible rack on top of the rice and place the lamb in the rack.
5. Put on the Pressure Lid and turn the pressure handle to the SEAL position.
6. Select Pressure Cook mode, set the pressure to High, and cooking time to 2 minutes. Hit the START/STOP button to initiate cooking.
7. Once it's done, release the pressure naturally, then remove the lid.
8. Add zucchini to the lamb and drizzle olive oil on top.
9. Put on the Crisping Lid and cook on GRILL mode for 10 minutes.
10. Serve the lamb with zucchini, rice, and lemon wedges

PORK CHOPS WITH APPLESAUCE

COOKING TIME: 24 MIN | SERVES 2

INGREDIENTS:

- 3 Golden apples, peeled and chopped
- Juice of ½ lemon
- 1 tsp. sugar
- ½ tsp. ground cinnamon
- ¼ tsp. salt
- 2 (12-oz.) boneless pork loin chops

- Cooking spray
- Black pepper, to taste

DIRECTIONS:

1. Mix apples with ½ cup water, lemon juice, salt, sugar, and cinnamon in the Ninja Foodi's insert.
2. Put on the Pressure Lid and turn the pressure handle to the SEAL position.
3. Select Pressure Cook mode, set the pressure to High, and cooking time to 4 minutes. Hit the START/STOP button to initiate cooking.
4. Once it's done, release the pressure quickly, then remove the lid.
5. Push the apples aside, place the reversible rack in the high position of Ninja Foodi's insert.
6. Coat the pork chops with cooking spray and rub them with black pepper and salt.
7. Place the seasoned pork chops in the reversible rack and put on the Crisping Lid.
8. Cook the chops on BROIL mode for 20 minutes.
9. Flip the chops once cooked halfway through, then resume cooking.
10. Transfer the chops to a serving plate.
11. Slightly mash the cooked apples in the pot and transfer them on top of the chops.
12. Serve warm.

MEATBALLS WITH CREAM SAUCE

COOKING TIME: 32 MIN | SERVES 6

INGREDIENTS:

- 17 ½ oz. ground beef and ground pork
- 1 onion, minced
- 2 tbsp. butter
- 2 garlic cloves, smashed
- 5 ¼ oz. chicken bouillon, heated
- 3 ½ fl. oz. water
- 1 egg

- 1 ½ oz. bread crumbs
- 1 tsp. paprika
- 1 tsp. oregano
- Salt and black pepper, to taste
- 1 tbsp. capers, chopped
- 1 jar capers

- 2 oz. flour
- 1 tbsp. wurze
- 1 bay leaf
- 1 tsp. parsley
- Juice 1/2 of lemon
- 14 oz. sour cream

DIRECTIONS:

1. Preheat the Ninja Foodi on SEAR/SAUTE mode at MD-HI for 5 minutes.
2. Add garlic, onions, and butter to the Ninja Foodi's insert and sauté for 5 minutes.
3. Mix ground beef with egg, ground pork, chopped capers, breadcrumbs, black pepper, oregano, salt, paprika, and sautéed garlic and onion in a bowl.
4. Make small meatballs out of this beef mixture and roll them in flour to coat.
5. Add drained capers from the jar to the Ninja Foodi's insert and sauté for 10 minutes.
6. Stir in meatballs and sauté for 15 minutes until brown.
7. Add lemon juice, wurze, bay leaf, white wine, and chicken bouillon.
8. Put on the Pressure Lid and turn the pressure handle to the SEAL position.
9. Select Pressure Cook mode, set the pressure to High, and cooking time to 12 minutes. Hit the START/STOP button to initiate cooking.
10. Once it's done, release the pressure naturally for 20 minutes, then remove the lid
11. Add sour cream and garnish with parsley.
12. Serve warm.

HERBED RACK OF LAMB

COOKING TIME: 35 MIN | SERVES 4

INGREDIENTS:

- 5 sprigs of fresh rosemary
- 1 (2½-lb.) rack of lamb, sliced in half
- Salt, to taste
- Black pepper, to taste

DIRECTIONS:

1. Rub the lamb with black pepper and salt, then place it in the Crisping Basket.
2. Place the rosemary sprigs on top of the lamb and transfer the basket to the Ninja Foodi's insert.
3. Put on the Crisping Lid and cook on AIR CRISP mode at 400 °F for 20 minutes.
4. Flip the chops and continue cooking on AIR CRISP mode for another 15 minutes.
5. Transfer the lamb to the cutting board and wrap it in a foil.
6. Leave the foil packed lamb for 10 minutes, then slice the rack into chops.
7. Chop the cooked rosemary and sprinkle over the lamb.
8. Serve warm.

MINT LAMB LEG

COOKING TIME: 43 MIN | SERVES 6

INGREDIENTS:

- ½ leg of lamb, raw
- 3 garlic cloves, peeled and sliced
- 1 small bunch fresh mint, sliced
- 2/3 oz. rapeseed oil
- Salt and black pepper, to taste
- 2/3 oz. thickening gravy granules

DIRECTIONS:

1. Carve small slits on top of the lamb leg and stuff slits with garlic, black pepper, and salt.
2. Add 7 oz cold water to the Ninja Foodi's insert and set the Crisping Basket inside.
3. Set the lamb leg in the reversible rack.
4. Put on the Pressure Lid and turn the pressure handle to the SEAL position.
5. Select Pressure Cook mode, set the pressure to High, and cooking time to 32 minutes. Hit the START/STOP button to initiate cooking.
6. Once it's done, release the pressure naturally, then remove the lid.
7. Brush the lamb with rapeseed oil and put on the Crisping Lid.
8. Cook on AIR CRISP mode at 395 °F for 8 minutes.
9. Transfer the lamb leg to a plate and cover it with a foil.
10. Add gravy granules to the cooking liquid and mix well.
11. Put on the Pressure Lid and turn the pressure handle to the SEAL position.
12. Select Pressure Cook mode, set the pressure to LOW, and cooking time to 3 minutes. Hit the START/STOP button to initiate cooking.
13. Once it's done, release the pressure naturally, then remove the lid.
14. Add mint to the sauce and pour over the lamb leg.
15. Serve warm.

BEEF CHEESEBURGERS

COOKING TIME: 28 MIN | SERVES 4

INGREDIENTS:

- 2 lbs. lean ground beef
- 2 tsp. salt
- 1 tsp. black pepper
- Cooking spray
- 6 bacon slices, cut in half crosswise
- 1½ cups cheddar cheese, shredded
- 4 burger buns, sliced in half

DIRECTIONS:

1. Mix beef with black pepper and salt in a bowl and make four patties out of it.
2. Set the reversible rack inside the Ninja Foodi's insert and grease it with cooking spray.
3. Spread the bacon slices in the rack and put on the Crisping Lid.
4. Select AIR CRISP mode, set time to 14 minutes, and temperature to 390 °F.
5. Flip the bacon and continue cooking for another 5 minutes. Transfer the crispy bacon to a plate lined with a paper towel.
6. Switch the Ninja Foodi to SEAR/SAUTE mode and heat the bacon fat for 5 minutes.
7. Add the burgers and sear them or 5 minutes per side.
8. Divide the cheddar cheese into four portions and flatten them into a round disk.
9. Place each cheese disk on top of the burger patties and put on the Crisping Lid.
10. Select BROIL mode and set the cooking time to 4 minutes, then press START/STOP.
11. Once the cheese is melted, transfer the burgers to the buns.
12. Serve warm.

ST. LOUIS PORK RIBS

COOKING TIME: 50 MIN | SERVES 6

INGREDIENTS:

- 1 tbsp. smoked paprika
- 1 tbsp. salt
- ½ tsp. black pepper
- 1 (2½-lb.) rack-style pork ribs
- ½ cup beer, light
- ½ cup apple cider vinegar
- 1 tsp. liquid smoke
- 1 cup Kansas-style barbecue sauce

DIRECTIONS:

1. Mix black pepper, salt, and paprika in a small bowl.
2. Rub this dry spice mix over the ribs rack.
3. Add liquid smoke, vinegar, and beer to the Ninja Foodi's insert.
4. Place the bracket stand from the Crisping Basket inside the Ninja Foodi's insert and set the ribs to rack in a position that it curls to make a cone.
5. Put on the Pressure Lid and turn the pressure handle to the SEAL position.
6. Select Pressure Cook mode, set the pressure to High, and cooking time to 20 minutes. Hit the START/STOP button to initiate cooking.
7. Once it's done, release the pressure naturally, then remove the lid.
8. Transfer the cooked ribs to a sheet pan and discard the liquid from the Ninja Foodi's insert.
9. Return the ribs to the Ninja Foodi, put on the Crisping Lid. Cook on AIR CRISP mode for 30 minutes at 400 °F.
10. Flip the rack after 10 minutes and brush it with BBQ sauce, then resume cooking.
11. Slice the ribs and serve warm.

PORK LETTUCE WRAPS

COOKING TIME: 55 MIN | SERVES 6

INGREDIENTS:

- 1 yellow onion, diced
- 7 garlic cloves, smashed
- 1 (3-inch) knob ginger, peeled and quartered
- 3 lbs. pork belly, skin removed
- 8 cups chicken stock
- 2 tsp. salt
- 1 tsp. black pepper
- Butter lettuce leaves (to garnish)
- Ssamjang (to garnish)
- Scallions, finely chopped (to garnish)

DIRECTIONS:

1. Add ginger, garlic, and onion to the Ninja Foodi's insert.
2. Place the Crisping Basket on top of this mixture and adjust the pork belly in the basket.
3. Drizzle black pepper and salt for seasoning and pour enough water to cover the pork.
4. Put on the Pressure Lid and turn the pressure handle to the SEAL position.
5. Select Pressure Cook mode, set the pressure to High, and cooking time to 35 minutes. Hit the START/STOP button to initiate cooking.
6. Once it's done, release the pressure naturally, then remove the lid.
7. Remove the basket from the Ninja Foodi, discard the cooking liquid and veggies.
8. Place the diffuser in the Ninja Foodi's insert and return the Crisping Basket.
9. Put on the Crisping Lid and cook on AIR CRISP mode for 20 minutes at 390 °F.
10. Once done, remove the pork belly and slice it after 10 minutes.
11. Divide the pork belly into lettuce leaves and garnish.
12. Serve warm.

CREAMY FILET MIGNON

COOKING TIME: 23 MIN | SERVES 2

INGREDIENTS:

- 1 lb. white potatoes, cubed
- 2 garlic cloves, smashed
- 2 (6-oz.) filet mignons
- Salt, to taste
- Black pepper, to taste
- Cooking spray
- 4 tbsp. butter, unsalted
- ½ cup heavy cream
- 2 sprigs fresh thyme

DIRECTIONS:

1. Add ½ cup water, garlic, and potatoes to the Ninja Foodi's insert.
2. Put on the Pressure Lid and turn the pressure handle to the SEAL position.
3. Select Pressure Cook mode, set the pressure to High, and cooking time to 3 minutes. Hit the START/STOP button to initiate cooking.
4. Once it's done, release the pressure naturally, then remove the lid.
5. Meanwhile, rub the filet Mignon with black pepper and salt.
6. Set the reversible rack in the high position of the Ninja Foodi's insert.
7. Place the filets in the rack and spray them with cooking spray. Put on the Crisping Lid and cook on BROIL mode for 10 minutes.
8. Flip the filets and drizzle cream and 2 tbsp butter over the filets. Resume cooking and BROIL for another 10 minutes.
9. Transfer the mignons to a plate and potatoes to a bowl.
10. Mash the soft potatoes with a masher and stir in ½ tsp salt. Mix well and serve the mignon with this potato mash.
11. Enjoy.

PORK SHOULDER WITH PINEAPPLE

COOKING TIME: 59 MIN | SERVES 6

INGREDIENTS:

- 1 (5 lbs.) boneless pork shoulder
- ½ pineapple, cored and cut into 6 strips
- ½ cup pineapple juice
- 6 dried guajillo chiles, stemmed and seeded
- 4 garlic cloves, smashed
- 2 tbsp. ground achiote
- 2 tbsp. cumin (ground)
- 2 tbsp. salt
- 1 tbsp. dried oregano
- Warmed corn tortillas (to garnish)
- White onion, finely diced (to garnish)
- Fresh cilantro, finely chopped (to garnish)
- Salsa (to garnish)

DIRECTIONS:

1. Cut the pork shoulder into 1-inch chunks.
2. Add pineapple strips, chiles, pineapple juice, achiote, garlic, oregano, salt, and cumin to the Ninja Foodi's insert.
3. Put on the Pressure Lid and turn the pressure handle to the SEAL position.
4. Select Pressure Cook mode, set the pressure to High, and cooking time to 4 minutes. Hit the START/STOP button to initiate cooking.
5. Once it's done, release the pressure naturally, then remove the lid.
6. Mash the pineapple sauce with a potato masher and add pork to this mash, then mix well.
7. Put on the Pressure Lid and turn the pressure handle to the SEAL position.
8. Select Pressure Cook mode, set the pressure to High, and cooking time to 45 minutes. Hit the START/STOP button to initiate cooking.
9. Once it's done, release the pressure naturally, then remove the lid.
10. Discard any excess liquid out of this pot and put on the Crisping Lid.
11. Cook on BROIL mode for 10 minutes.
12. Divide the pork mixture into tortillas and garnish with salsa, cilantro, and onion.
13. Serve warm.

BBQ RIBS

COOKING TIME: 40 MIN | SERVES 4

INGREDIENTS:

- 18 oz. barbecue sauce
- 3 ½ lbs. rack of ribs
- ½ cup apple cider

DIRECTIONS:

1. Remove the membranes from the ribs rack.
2. Place the rib rack in the Ninja Foodi's insert with its meat side up and brush its top with barbecue sauce.
3. Pour apple cider over the rack of ribs.
4. Put on the Pressure Lid and turn the pressure handle to the SEAL position.
5. Select Pressure Cook mode, set the pressure to High, and cooking time to 30 minutes. Hit the START/STOP button to initiate cooking.
6. Once it's done, release the pressure naturally for 5 minutes, then remove the lid.
7. Transfer the ribs to a cutting board, slice it, and pour its sauce into a bowl.
8. Set a reversible rack in the Ninja Foodi's insert and add 2 pork pieces on the rack.
9. Pour some sauce over the ribs and put on the Crisping Lid. Cook on AIR CRISP mode for 10 minutes at 400 °F.
10. Repeat the same process with the remaining ribs and sauce.
11. Serve warm.

CHUCK ROAST WITH GRAVY

COOKING TIME: 87 MIN | SERVES 6

INGREDIENTS:

- 4 lbs. boneless chuck roast
- 1 pinch salt
- 1 pinch black pepper
- 1 tbsp. olive oil
- 1 cup onion, chopped
- 1 tbsp. garlic, minced
- ¼ cup tomato sauce
- ¼ cup red wine
- 3 cups beef broth
- 1 tbsp. Worcestershire sauce
- 1 tbsp. dried thyme
- 1 tbsp. dried rosemary
- 1 bay leaf
- 4-8 oz. mushrooms, sliced
- 1 lb. red potatoes, cut in half
- 1 lb. carrots, peeled and cut in half
- Corn starch slurry
- 3 tbsp. corn starch
- 6 tbsp. water (cold)

DIRECTIONS:

1. Dice the chuck roast into 4x4 inches pieces.
2. Add 1 tbsp olive to the Ninja Foodi's insert and heat it on SEAR/SAUTE mode on HI.
3. Stir in chuck roast cubes and sauté for 10 minutes until they are brown, then transfer them to a plate.
4. Add chopped onion and sauté for about 3 minutes. Stir in tomato paste, red wine, and garlic, then cook for 1 minute.
5. Add beef broth, rosemary, thyme, and Worcestershire sauce. Mix well and add the sautéed chuck roast and bay leaf.
6. Put on the Pressure Lid and turn the pressure handle to the SEAL position.
7. Select Pressure Cook mode, set the pressure to High, and cooking time to 65 minutes. Hit the START/STOP button to initiate cooking.
8. Once it's done, release the pressure naturally for 15, then remove the lid. Remove the roast from the pot and place it on a plate.
9. Add mushrooms, potatoes, and carrots to the Ninja Foodi's insert.
10. Put on the Pressure Lid and turn the pressure handle to the SEAL position.
11. Select Pressure Cook mode, set the pressure to High, and cooking time to 5 minutes. Hit the START/STOP button to initiate cooking.
12. Once it's done, release the pressure naturally, then remove the lid.
13. Mix cornstarch with water in a small glass bowl and pour into the Ninja Foodi's insert.
14. Switch the Ninja Foodi to SEAR/SAUTE mode and cook for 3 minutes with occasional stirring.
15. Return the roast to the gravy and mix well.
16. Serve warm.

BEEF BURGERS

COOKING TIME: 13 MIN | SERVES 8

INGREDIENTS:

- 1 tbsp. avocado oil
- 3 tbsp. dark brown sugar
- 1 tsp. dry mustard
- 1 ½ lb. lean ground beef
- 1 cup onion, diced
- 1 tbsp. Worcestershire sauce
- 1 cup red bell pepper, diced

- 1 tbsp. chili powder
- 1 ½ tsp. garlic, diced
- 1 ½ cups tomatoes, crushed and drained
- ¼ cup apple cider vinegar
- 8 hamburger buns
- ¼ cup water
- 4 tbsp. butter

- 1 tsp. salt
- 1 pinch red pepper flakes
- Black pepper, to taste

DIRECTIONS:

1. Add oil to the Ninja Foodi's insert and heat it on SEAR/SAUTE mode.
2. Stir in red bell pepper, ground beef, and onion, then sauté for 7 minutes. Add garlic and sauté for 30 seconds.
3. Stir in water, brown sugar, vinegar, chili powder, mustard, Worcestershire sauce, red pepper flakes, and tomato paste.
4. Stir in crushed tomatoes, salt, and black pepper, then mix well.
5. Put on the Pressure Lid and turn the pressure handle to the SEAL position.
6. Select Pressure Cook mode, set the pressure to High, and cooking time to 5 minutes. Hit the START/STOP button to initiate cooking.
7. Once it's done, release the pressure naturally for 10 minutes, then remove the lid.
8. Toast buns in butter in a hot skillet. Divide the beef in between two halves of the buns.
9. Serve warm

CHINESE BBQ PORK WITH POTATOES

COOKING TIME: 19 MIN | SERVES 4

INGREDIENTS:

- 3 sweet potatoes, peeled and cubed
- ½ cup coconut milk, unsweetened
- 4 frozen boneless pork chops
- ¼ cup hoisin sauce
- 1/3 cup honey
- 1 ½ tbsp. soy sauce
- 1 tsp. Chinese five-spice powder

- ½ stick butter
- 1 tbsp. ginger, minced
- Salt, to taste
- ½ tsp. white pepper

DIRECTIONS:

1. Add coconut milk and potatoes to the Ninja Foodi's insert.
2. Set the reversible rack over it and set the pork chops in the rack.
3. Put on the Pressure Lid and turn the pressure handle to the SEAL position.
4. Select Pressure Cook mode, set the pressure to High, and cooking time to 4 minutes. Hit the START/STOP button to initiate cooking.
5. Once it's done, release the pressure naturally, then remove the lid.
6. Mix hoisin sauce with Chinese five-spice, soy sauce, and honey in a bowl.
7. Transfer the ribs to a plate, and mix potatoes with ginger, salt, and butter in a bowl.
8. Mash the soft potatoes with a fork and mix well.
9. Return the rack to the Ninja Foodi's insert and place the chops in it.
10. Brush the chops with ½ of the prepared sauce, then close the lid.
11. Cook on BROIL Mode for 15 minutes and baste the chops with remaining sauce once cooked halfway through.
12. Serve the chops with mashed potatoes.

MEATBALLS WITH SPAGHETTI

COOKING TIME: 24 MIN | SERVES 4

INGREDIENTS:

Meatballs:
- 2 lbs. lean ground beef
- 1 cup Italian breadcrumbs
- ¼ cup milk
- ¼ cup Parmesan cheese, shredded
- 1 large egg, beaten
- 8 fresh basil leaves, minced
- 4 garlic cloves, smashed

- 2½ tsp. salt
- 1 tsp. red pepper flakes
- Cooking spray

Sauce and Spaghetti:
- 1 yellow onion, diced
- 3 garlic cloves, smashed
- 5 fresh basil leaves

- 2 tbsp. olive oil
- 1 tsp. salt
- 4 tbsp. butter, unsalted
- 1 (1-lb.) box spaghetti
- 4 cups tomato sauce

DIRECTIONS:

1. Mix beef with milk, garlic, red pepper flakes, salt, egg, basil, Parmesan, and breadcrumbs in a bowl.
2. Make 8 meatballs out of this mixture and keep them aside.
3. Set a Crisping Basket inside the Ninja Foodi's insert and grease it with cooking spray.
4. Place the meatballs in the basket, coat them with cooking spray and cover with a Crisping Lid.
5. Cook on BROIL mode for 20 minutes, then transfer the meatballs to a plate.
6. Empty the pot and switch the Ninja Foodi to SEAR/SAUTE mode on High.
7. Stir in olive oil, basil, salt, garlic, and onion, then sauté for 4 minutes. Stir in pasta and 2 ¼ cups water.
8. Put on the Pressure Lid and turn the pressure handle to the SEAL position.
9. Select Pressure Cook mode, set the pressure to High, and cooking time to 0 minutes. Hit the START/STOP button to initiate cooking.
10. Once it's done, release the pressure naturally for 12 minutes, then remove the lid.
11. Add tomato sauce, ½ cup water, and butter, then mix well.
12. Put on the Pressure Lid and turn the pressure handle to the SEAL position.
13. Select Pressure Cook mode, set the pressure to High, and cooking time to 0 minutes. Hit the START/STOP button to initiate cooking.
14. Once it's done, release the pressure quickly, then remove the lid. Add meatballs to the pasta and sauce, then mix well.
15. Serve warm.

PANCETTA PASTA CARBONARA

COOKING TIME: 32 MIN | SERVES 4

INGREDIENTS:

- 4 oz. pancetta, diced
- 1 (1 lb.) box spaghetti
- 4 large egg yolks

- ½ cup pecorino cheese, finely grated
- ½ cup Parmesan cheese, finely grated
- Salt, to taste

DIRECTIONS:

1. Sauté pancetta in the Ninja Foodi's insert on SEAR/SAUTE mode for 8 minutes.
2. Transfer the crispy pancetta to a plate.
3. Add spaghetti and 3 cups of water to the same Ninja Foodi's insert.
4. Put on the Pressure Lid and turn the pressure handle to the SEAL position.
5. Select Pressure Cook mode, set the pressure to High, and cooking time to 32 minutes. Hit the START/STOP button to initiate cooking.
6. Once it's done, release the pressure naturally for 12 minutes, then remove the lid.
7. Beat egg yolks with ½ cup water and cheeses in a bowl.
8. Return the pancetta to the Ninja Foodi and mix well.
9. Slowly pour in the egg mixture and mix well until it is incorporated, then adjust seasoning with salt.
10. Serve warm.

BBQ MEATLOAF

COOKING TIME: 30 MIN | SERVES 8

INGREDIENTS:

- 1 lb. ground beef
- ¼ cup cilantro leaves
- ¼ cup barbecue sauce, divided
- 1 cup of water
- 1 cup corn chips, crushed
- 1 egg

- 1 bell pepper, diced
- ½ jalapeño pepper, deseeded, minced
- 1 onion, peeled and diced
- 3 corn tortillas, chopped
- 1 tbsp. garlic powder
- 2 tsp. cumin (ground)

- 2 tsp. chili powder
- 1 tsp. cayenne pepper
- Salt, to taste

DIRECTIONS:

1. Mix beef with tortillas, bell peppers, jalapeno pepper, cilantro, spices, onion, and barbecue sauce in a suitable baking pan.
2. Cover this pan with a foil sheet.
3. Add water to the Ninja Foodi's insert and set a trivet inside, then place the pan on it.
4. Put on the Pressure Lid and turn the pressure handle to the SEAL position.
5. Select Pressure Cook mode, set the pressure to High, and cooking time to 15 minutes. Hit the START/STOP button to initiate cooking.
6. Once it's done, release the pressure quickly, then remove the lid.
7. Remove the foil from the pan and cover the lid again.
8. Now switch the Ninja Foodi to BAKE/ROAST mode and cook for 15 minutes at 360 °F.
9. After 7 minutes, mix corn chips with 2 tbsp barbeque sauce and spread over the meatloaf. Resume cooking for the remaining 8 minutes.
10. Slice and serve warm.

BEEF RICOTTA LASAGNA

COOKING TIME: 69 MIN | SERVES 6

INGREDIENTS:

- 2¼ lbs. lean ground beef
- 2 tsp. salt
- 1 yellow onion, diced
- 4 garlic cloves, smashed
- 3 whole fresh basil leaves
- 1 (33 oz.) can tomato sauce
- 1 large egg

- 1 (15-oz.) container ricotta
- 1 (1-lb.) package mozzarella cheese, shredded
- 2 tsp. dried oregano
- Black pepper, to taste
- 1 (12-oz.) box oven-ready lasagna noodles

DIRECTIONS:

1. Sauté beef with 2 tsp salt in the Ninja Foodi's insert on SEAR/SAUTE mode for 10 minutes. Transfer this meat to a plate.
2. Add basil, garlic, and onion to the same pot and sauté for 7 minutes.
3. Stir in tomato sauce and sautéed meat, then mix well. Transfer it to a bow.
4. Beat egg with ricotta, black pepper, salt, and oregano.
5. Spread 2 cups of the meat sauce at the base of Ninja Foodi's insert.
6. Top the sauce with 3 lasagna noodles spread in a single layer.
7. Spread the 1/3 ricotta mixture on top of the lasagna. Repeat these layers to use the remaining meat sauce, noodles, and ricotta mixture.
8. Pour ½ cup water around these layers and drizzle mozzarella cheese on top.
9. Put on the Pressure Lid and turn the pressure handle to the VENT position.
10. Select STEAM mode, and set the cooking time to 45 minutes. Hit the START/STOP button to initiate cooking.
11. Once it's done, release the pressure quickly, then remove the lid.
12. Put on the Crisping Lid and cook on BROIL mode for 7 minutes.
13. Serve warm.

SAUSAGE RIGATONI PASTA

COOKING TIME: 23 MIN | SERVES 8

INGREDIENTS:

- 1 lb. Italian Sausage
- 1 large onion, diced
- 1 tsp. salt
- 1/2 tsp. dried oregano
- 1/2 tsp. dried basil
- 1/4 tsp. black pepper

- 1/4 tsp. crushed red pepper
- 6 large cloves garlic, minced or pressed
- 1 cup red wine
- 1 can (28 oz.) peeled San Marzano tomatoes
- 1 can (28 oz.) San Marzano tomato puree
- 2 cups chicken stock

- 1 (16 oz.) box dry rigatoni pasta
- 4 cups mozzarella, shredded
- 1 package (6 oz.) pepperoni, thin-sliced

DIRECTIONS:

1. Preheat your Ninja Foodi on SEAR/SAUTE mode on MD: HI for 5 minutes.
2. Add sausage and sauté until brown. Transfer and crumble the bacon onto a plate.
3. Sauté onion with olive oil in the Ninja Foodi's insert for 2 minutes.
4. Stir in red pepper, black pepper, basil, oregano, and salt, then sauté for 5 minutes.
5. Add garlic, wine, browned sausage, tomatoes, pasta, chicken stock, and tomato puree.
6. Put on the Pressure Lid and turn the pressure handle to the SEAL position.
7. Select Pressure Cook mode, set the pressure to High, and cooking time to 6 minutes. Hit the START/STOP button to initiate cooking.
8. Once it's done, release the pressure naturally for 10 minutes, then remove the lid.
9. Mix the pasta with the sauce, then top it with 3 cups mozzarella and pepperoni slices.
10. Add remaining mozzarella on top and put on the Crisping Lid.
11. Cook on AIR CRISP mode for 5 minutes at 400 °F.
12. Serve warm.

BEEF CHILI CASSEROLE

COOKING TIME: 49 MIN | SERVES 8

INGREDIENTS:

- 2 lbs. ground beef, uncooked
- 14 oz. kidney beans, rinsed, drained
- 28 oz. crushed tomatoes
- 1 cup beef stock
- 2 cups Cheddar Cornbread batter, uncooked
- 1 cup Mexican cheese blend, shredded
- 1 onion, peeled and diced

- 1 bell pepper, diced
- 1 jalapeño pepper, diced, deseeded
- 4 garlic cloves, peeled and minced
- 2 tbsp. cumin (ground)
- 1 tbsp. onion powder
- 1 tbsp. garlic powder
- Salt, to taste

- black pepper, to taste
- Sour cream (to garnish)

DIRECTIONS:

1. Mix beef with tomatoes, stock, and beans to the Ninja Foodi's insert.
2. Put on the Pressure Lid and turn the pressure handle to the SEAL position.
3. Select Pressure Cook mode, set the pressure to High, and cooking time to 15 minutes. Hit the START/STOP button to initiate cooking.
4. Once it's done, release the pressure quickly, then remove the lid.
5. Add bell peppers, onions, garlic, jalapeno pepper, cumin, garlic powder, and onion powder.
6. Switch the Ninja Foodi to SEAR/SAUTE mode and cook for 5 minutes.
7. Spread the cheddar corn batter on top and cover the lid.
8. Cook on BAKE/ROAST mode for 26 minutes at 360 °F. Drizzle cheese on top put on the Crisping Lid, and BROIL for 3 minutes.
9. Garnish with cream. Serve warm.

VEGETARIAN

CHEESY MACARONI BAKE

COOKING TIME: 12 MIN | SERVES 8

INGREDIENTS:

- 71 tbsp. baking soda
- ½ cup fresh lemon juice
- 1 lb. elbow macaroni
- 1 cup heavy cream
- 4 cups cheddar cheese, shredded
- 1 tbsp. salt
- 1 tbsp. black pepper
- 1 tbsp. onion powder
- 1 tbsp. garlic powder
- 1 tsp. dry mustard
- 2 cups panko breadcrumbs
- ½ cup (1 stick) butter, unsalted, melted

DIRECTIONS:

1. Mix lemon juice with baking soda in the Ninja Foodi's insert.
2. Add 5 cups water and macaroni, then mix well.
3. Put on the Pressure Lid and turn the pressure handle to the SEAL position.
4. Select Pressure Cook mode, set the pressure to LOW, and cooking time to 5 minutes. Hit the START/STOP button to initiate cooking.
5. Once it's done, release the pressure naturally for 10 minutes, then remove the lid.
6. Add cheese, cream, onion, garlic powder, black pepper, salt, and dry mustard.
7. Mix well then allow the cheese to melt.
8. Toss breadcrumbs with melted butter in a bowl and spread on top of macaroni.
9. Put on the Crisping Lid and cook AIR CRISP mode for 7 minutes at 390 °F.
10. Serve warm.

CHILI MAC & CHEESE

COOKING TIME: 2 MIN | SERVES 6

INGREDIENTS:

- 1 (1 lb.) box elbow macaroni
- 3 tbsp. butter, unsalted
- ¾ cup heavy cream
- 2 large eggs
- 1 tsp. dry mustard
- 1½ tsp. salt
- 1 small red chilli, chopped
- 10 oz. mild cheddar cheese, shredded
- Black pepper, to taste

DIRECTIONS:

1. Add macaroni to the Ninja Foodi's insert and pour enough water to cover it.
2. Put on the Pressure Lid and turn the pressure handle to the SEAL position.
3. Select Pressure Cook mode, set the pressure to High, and cooking time to 0 minutes. Hit the START/STOP button to initiate cooking.
4. Once it's done, release the pressure naturally for 12 minutes, then remove the lid.
5. Add butter and chopped chilli to the macaroni and mix well.
6. Beat eggs with mustard, cream, and salt in a suitable bowl.
7. Switch the Ninja Foodi to SEAR/SAUTE mode and pour in the egg mixture.
8. Add cheese and cook for 2 minutes with occasional stirring.
9. Garnish with black pepper.
10. Serve warm.

PARMESAN PUMPKIN RISOTTO

COOKING TIME: 10 MIN | SERVES 4

INGREDIENTS:

- 4 tbsp. butter
- 8.5 oz. arborio rice
- 4 ½ cups vegetable broth
- 2 tbsp. olive oil
- 1 onion, diced
- 1 garlic clove, minced
- 1 ½ cups pumpkin, diced
- 2 tsp. salt
- Black pepper, to taste
- 1/2 cup grated parmesan cheese
- 2 tsp. parsley, chopped
- 4 tsp. Parmesan, shaved
- 1 tbsp. cream

DIRECTIONS:

1. Sauté onion with olive oil and butter in Ninja Foodi's insert on SEAR/SAUTE mode for 3 minutes.
2. Toss in pumpkin cubes and sauté for 2 minutes.
3. Stir in rice, 1 tsp salt, and broth, then mix them well.
4. Put on the Pressure Lid and turn the pressure handle to the SEAL position.
5. Select Pressure Cook mode, set the pressure to High, and cooking time to 7 minutes. Hit the START/STOP button to initiate cooking.
6. Once it's done, release the pressure naturally, then remove the lid.
7. Switch the Ninja Foodi to SEAR/SAUTE mode and add parmesan cheese and butter to the risotto.
8. Mix well and garnish with parsley, parmesan shavings and cream.
9. Serve warm.

SPICED CHICKPEA FRY

COOK TIME: 50 MINS | SERVES 4

INGREDIENTS:

- 1 can chickpeas
- ¼ tsp. allspice
- ¼ tsp. cinnamon
- ¼ tsp. smoked paprika
- ¼ tsp. ginger (ground)
- ½ tsp. coriander (ground)
- ½ tsp. turmeric (ground)
- ½ tbsp. cumin (ground)
- ¼ tsp. of salt
- 1 pinch cayenne pepper
- 1 pinch black pepper
- Cooking sprays

DIRECTIONS:

1. Rinse the chickpeas in a sieve and transfer them to a bowl.
2. Add spices and mix well. Then coat the chickpeas with cooking spray.
3. Spread these chickpeas in the Ninja Foodi's Crisping Basket and place the basket in the Ninja Foodi's insert.
4. Put on Crisping Lid and cook on AIR CRISP mode for 20 minutes.
5. Serve warm.

JAPANESE MUSHROOM CURRY

COOKING TIME: 6 MIN | SERVES 6

INGREDIENTS:

- 4 carrots, chopped
- 4 parsnips, chopped
- 1 lb. fresh button mushrooms, sliced
- 2 russet potatoes, peeled and chopped
- ½ yellow onion, chopped
- 1 (8.4-oz.) package Japanese curry bricks
- Steamed rice (to serve)

DIRECTIONS:

1. Add 6 cups water, onion, potatoes, mushrooms, parsnips, and carrots to the Ninja Foodi's insert.
2. Put on the Pressure Lid and turn the pressure handle to the SEAL position.
3. Select Pressure Cook mode set the pressure to High and cooking time to 3 minutes. Hit the START/STOP button to initiate cooking.
4. Once it's done, release the pressure quickly, then remove the lid.
5. Switch the Ninja foodi to SEAR/SAUTE mode on High.
6. Stir in curry bricks and cook for 3 minutes with constant stirring.
7. Serve warm with rice.

CHICKPEA SPINACH STEW

COOKING TIME: 42 MIN | SERVES 6

INGREDIENTS:

- 2 cups dried chickpeas
- 2 tsp. salt
- 3 tbsp. ghee
- 1 yellow onion, diced
- 2 garlic cloves, minced
- 1-inch knob ginger, peeled and minced
- 2 tsp. garam masala
- 1 tsp. cumin (ground)
- ½ tsp. cayenne
- ½ tsp. turmeric (ground)
- 2 plum tomatoes, seeded and diced
- 20 oz. fresh baby spinach, chopped
- 1 cup evaporated milk
- Finely chopped fresh cilantro (to garnish)
- Steamed basmati rice (to serve)

DIRECTIONS:

1. Add 5 cups water, ½ tsp salt, and chickpeas to Ninja Foodi's insert.
2. Put on the Pressure Lid and turn the pressure handle to the SEAL position.
3. Select Pressure Cook mode set the pressure to High and cooking time to 30 minutes. Hit the START/STOP button to initiate cooking.
4. Once it's done, release the pressure naturally for 15 minutes, then remove the lid.
5. Drain the chickpeas and empty the Ninja Foodi's insert.
6. Switch the Ninja foodi to SEAR/SAUTE mode on High.
7. Stir in ghee, garlic, ginger, and onion, then sauté for 6 minutes.
8. Add turmeric, cayenne, cumin, garam masala, and remaining salt.
9. Sauté for 1 minute, then add chickpeas, tomatoes, spinach, and pour in evaporated milk.
10. Cook for 5 minutes with occasional stirring.
11. Garnish with cilantro and serve warm with rice.

BEAN BURGERS

COOKING TIME: 13 MIN | SERVES 4

INGREDIENTS:

- 2 cups refried black beans
- 1 cup panko breadcrumbs
- 2 tbsp. vegetable shortening
- 1 tsp. soy sauce
- 1 tsp. vegan Worcestershire sauce
- 3 drops liquid smoke
- ¼ tsp. dry mustard
- Cooking spray
- 4 burger buns

DIRECTIONS:

1. Toss refried beans with soy sauce, shortening, breadcrumbs, liquid smoke, Worcestershire sauce, and mustard in a bowl.
2. Mash this mixture and make 4 patties out of it. Place the patties in a plate and cover to refrigerate for 1 hour or more.
3. Preheat the Ninja Foodi's insert on SEAR/SAUTE mode on High for 5 minutes.
4. Grease it with cooking spray and sear the patties for 4 minutes per side.
5. Serve the patties in the buns.
6. Enjoy.

CHEESY ZUCCHINI QUICHE

COOKING TIME: 40 MIN | SERVES 6

INGREDIENTS:

- 3 eggs
- 2 medium zucchinis, sliced
- 1 onion, chopped
- 1 cup mozzarella, shredded
- 15 oz. half-skimmed ricotta
- ½ tsp. dried basil
- 1 tbsp. butter
- ½ tsp. dried oregano
- Cooking spray
- Black pepper, a dash

DIRECTIONS:

1. Preheat the Ninja Foodi's insert on SEAR/SAUTE mode.
2. Add butter and zucchini, then sauté for 5 minutes.
3. Stir in onions and sauté for 5 minutes.
4. Add peppers and seasoning, then mix well. Switch off the Ninja foodi.
5. Beat eggs with mozzarella and ricotta cheese in a casserole dish.
6. Stir in zucchini and onion mixture, then mix gently.
7. Add 1 cup water to the Ninja Foodi's insert and set a trivet inside.
8. Place the casserole dish over this trivet.
9. Put on the Pressure Lid and turn the pressure handle to the SEAL position.
10. Select Pressure Cook mode set the pressure to High and cooking time to 30 minutes. Hit the START/STOP button to initiate cooking.
11. Once it's done, release the pressure naturally, then remove the lid.
12. Serve warm.

ZITI CHEESE BAKE

COOKING TIME: 6 MIN | SERVES 8

INGREDIENTS:

- 71 (1-lb.) package ziti
- 1 yellow onion, diced
- 4 garlic cloves, minced
- 4 fresh basil leaves, minced
- 1 tbsp. soy sauce
- 1 tbsp. sugar

- 1 tbsp. dried oregano
- 1 tsp. red pepper flakes
- 2 tsp. salt
- 1 (16-oz.) can tomato sauce
- 4 cups mozzarella, shredded
- ½ cup Parmesan cheese, grated

- Black pepper, to taste

DIRECTIONS:

1. Add 2 ½ cup water, ziti, onion, soy sauce, basil, garlic, oregano, sugar, salt, and red pepper flakes to the Ninja Foodi's insert.
2. Put on the Pressure Lid and turn the pressure handle to the SEAL position.
3. Select Pressure Cook mode set the pressure to High and cooking time to 0 minutes. Hit the START/STOP button to initiate cooking.
4. Once it's done, release the pressure naturally, then remove the lid.
5. Add tomato sauce, parmesan, ½ cup water, and 2 cups mozzarella to the pot.
6. Put on the Pressure Lid and turn the pressure handle to the SEAL position.
7. Select Pressure Cook mode set the pressure to High and cooking time to 0 minutes. Hit the START/STOP button to initiate cooking.
8. Once it's done, release the pressure quickly, then remove the lid.
9. Stir in the remaining 2 cups of mozzarella cheese and put on the crisping lid.
10. Cook for 6 minutes on BROIL mode.
11. Garnish with black pepper and grated parmesan and serve warm

INDIAN KIDNEY BEAN CURRY

COOKING TIME: 49 MIN | SERVES 4

INGREDIENTS:

- 1 tbsp. ghee
- 1 tsp. cumin seeds
- 2 green chilies, pierced
- 1 onion, diced
- 1-inch ginger, grated
- 6 garlic cloves, crushed
- 9 oz. passata

- 18 oz. water
- ½ tsp. turmeric powder
- 1 ½ tsp. cumin powder
- 1 tsp. coriander powder
- 1 tsp. red chili powder
- 1 tsp. salt
- ¼ tsp. black pepper

- 6 ½ oz. red kidney beans (soaked overnight)
- 1 tsp. garam masala
- 1 tsp. madras curry powder

DIRECTIONS:

1. Melt ghee in the Ninja Foodi's insert on SEAR/SAUTE mode on MD: HI for 5 minutes.
2. Stir in green chilies, and cumin seeds then sauté for 1 minute.
3. Toss in onions and sauté for 7 minutes until golden.
4. Stir in garlic and ginger, then sauté for 30 seconds.
5. Stir in beans and the rest of the ingredients except curry powder and garam masala.
6. Put on the Pressure Lid and turn the pressure handle to the SEAL position.
7. Select Pressure Cook mode set the pressure to High and cooking time to 30 minutes. Hit the START/STOP button to initiate cooking.
8. Once it's done, release the pressure naturally, then remove the lid.
9. Stir in curry powder and garam masala then mix well.
10. Switch the Ninja Foodi to SEAR/SAUTE mode and cook for 5 minutes.
11. Serve warm.

BROCCOLI RICE NOODLES

COOKING TIME: 26 MIN | SERVES 4

INGREDIENTS:

- 1 (14-oz.) package rice noodles
- ¼ cup vegetable oil
- 2 tbsp. 1 tsp. oyster sauce
- 1 tbsp. light soy sauce
- 1 tbsp. sugar
- 1 tbsp. rice vinegar
- 1 garlic clove, minced
- 12 oz. fresh broccoli florets, split
- 2 large eggs
- 3 tbsp. sweet, dark soy sauce

DIRECTIONS:

1. Plug in the instant pot and grease the stainless steel insert with olive oil. Press the "Sauté" button and add onions. Stir-fry until translucent. Now, add beef and tomato paste. Continue to cook for 5 more minutes, stirring occasionally.
2. Meanwhile, whisk together eggs, milk, goat's cheese, rosemary powder, garlic powder, and salt. Pour the mixture into the pot and stir slowly with a wooden spatula. Cook until slightly underdone.
3. Remove from the heat and serve.

VEGETABLE JAPCHAE NOODLES

COOKING TIME: 40 MIN | SERVES 4

INGREDIENTS:

- 7 oz ground beef
- 1 (8-oz.) package japchae noodles
- Cooking spray
- 2 large egg yolks, beaten
- 2 tbsp. vegetable oil
- 2 tbsp. 1 tsp. toasted sesame oil
- 2 carrots, shredded
- 8 oz. button mushrooms, sliced
- ½ red bell pepper, seeded, and sliced
- ½ yellow onion, sliced
- ¼ cup soy sauce
- 2 tbsp. sugar
- 1 tbsp. toasted sesame seeds
- 2 cups baby spinach
- 1 tsp. salt
- ½ tsp. black pepper
- Sliced scallions (to garnish)

DIRECTIONS:

1. Add noodles to the Ninja Foodi's crisping basket and set it inside the Ninja Foodi's insert.
2. Pour water into the Ninja Foodi's insert to reach up to the fill line.
3. Switch the Ninja foodi to SEAR/SAUTE on High and cook for 15 minutes.
4. Remove the noodles, and the basket then drain the noodles in a colander.
5. Empty the pot and grease it with cooking spray.
6. Heat the Ninja Foodi's insert on SEAR/SAUTE mode on high for 3 minutes.
7. Pour in egg yolks and cook for 1 minute then flip and cook for 1 minute. Transfer the egg yolk to a plate and chop it.
8. Add vegetable oil and 1 tsp sesame oil to the Ninja Foodi's insert.
9. Stir in onion, bell pepper, mushrooms and carrots then toss well.
10. Put on the crisping lid and cook on AIR CRISP mode at 390 °F for 12 minutes.
11. Mix soy sauce, sesame seeds, sugar, and 2 tbsp sesame oil in a bowl.
12. Add noodles and soy sauce mixture to the veggies and mix well.
13. Stir in spinach and cooked egg yolks.
14. Put on the crisping lid and cook on AIR CRISP mode for 10 minutes at 390 °F.
15. Garnish with scallions and serve.

PASTA PEPPER SALAD

COOKING TIME: 3 MIN | SERVES 6

INGREDIENTS:

- 4 cups of water
- 16 oz. elbow pasta
- 2 tbsp. olive oil
- ½ cup red onion, diced
- ¼ cup black olives
- 1 cup roasted red peppers, sliced
- ½ lb. fresh mozzarella, diced
- ½ cup basil, chopped
- 1 tbsp. salt

DIRECTIONS:

1. Add pasta, water, and salt to the Ninja Foodi's insert.
2. Put on the Pressure Lid and turn the pressure handle to the SEAL position.
3. Select Pressure Cook mode set the pressure to High and cooking time to 3 minutes. Hit the START/STOP button to initiate cooking.
4. Once it's done, release the pressure naturally, then remove the lid.
5. Drain the pasta and transfer to a salad bowl.
6. Toss in 2 tbsp oil, red onion, basil, black olives, roasted peppers, and mozzarella.
7. Mix well and serve.

CRUSTED EGGPLANT PARMESAN

COOKING TIME: 55 MIN | SERVES 4

INGREDIENTS:

- 1 tbsp. garlic infused oil
- 1 tbsp. ginger, grated
- 1 red chili, diced
- 1 red pepper, julienned
- 2 tbsp. fresh chives, chopped
- 1 2/3 oz. baby corn, sliced
- 1 large handful of beansprouts
- 10 ½ oz. vermicelli rice noodles
- 1 medium carrot, julienned
- 1 medium courgette, julienned
- 1 large handful spring greens, shredded
- 4 tsp. curry powder
- 1/2 tbsp. maple syrup
- 3 tbsp. tamari
- Juice of 1 lime
- 2 lime wedges (to garnish)
- 2 tbsp. fresh chopped coriander (to garnish)

DIRECTIONS:

1. Place the eggplant slices in the Ninja Foodi's crisping basket and set the lemon on top.
2. Insert the basket back into the Ninja Foodi's insert and pour 1 cup water in it.
3. Put on the Pressure Lid and turn the pressure handle to the SEAL position.
4. Select Pressure Cook mode set the pressure to High and cooking time to 0 minutes. Hit the START/STOP button to initiate cooking.
5. Once it's done, release the pressure quickly, then remove the lid.
6. Remove the eggplants and empty the pot. Pat dry the cooked eggplants.
7. Beat eggs in one bowl and mix breadcrumbs with panko in another bowl.
8. Dip each eggplant slice in the eggs, then coat them with breadcrumbs mixture.
9. Return the slices to the Ninja Foodi's crisping basket and insert it into the Ninja Foodi's insert. Spray the slices with cooking spray.
10. Put on the crisping lid and cook on AIR CRISP Mode for 30 minutes.
11. Flip the slices and cook for another 20 minutes.
12. Empty the Ninja Foodi's insert and place the eggplant slices in it.
13. Add marinara sauce and cheese on top.
14. Put on the crisping lid and cook on BROIL Mode for 5 minutes.
15. Serve warm.

SWEET POTATO BEAN TACOS

COOKING TIME: 71 MIN | SERVES 8

INGREDIENTS:

- 1 lb. dried black beans, rinsed
- 2 chipotle chiles in adobo sauce
- 2 garlic cloves, minced
- 1 tsp. cumin (ground)
- 1 tsp. salt
- ½ tsp. coriander (ground)
- Sweet Potatoes

- 3 tbsp. vegetable oil
- 1 tbsp. sauce from chipotles in adobo sauce
- 2 tsp. cumin (ground)
- 1 tsp. salt
- 3 sweet potatoes, peeled and diced
- 20 (6-inch) corn tortillas, warmed
- Sour cream (to garnish)

- Salsa or Pico de Gallo (to garnish)
- Mexican-style cheese, shredded (to garnish)
- Chopped fresh cilantro (to garnish)

DIRECTIONS:

1. Add black beans, garlic, chili, salt, 6 cups water and coriander to the Ninja Foodi's insert.
2. Put on the Pressure Lid and turn the pressure handle to the SEAL position.
3. Select Pressure Cook mode set the pressure to High and cooking time to 25 minutes. Hit the START/STOP button to initiate cooking.
4. Once it's done, release the pressure naturally, then remove the lid.
5. Transfer the beans to a bowl and allow them to cool.
6. Sauté adobo sauce, cumin, salt with oil in the Ninja Foodi's insert on SEAR/SAUTE mode for 1 minute.
7. Stir in sweet potatoes and sauté for 1 minute.
8. Put on the crisping lid and cook on AIR CRISP Mode for 45 minutes at 390 °F.
9. Divide the beans and potatoes in the warm tortillas.
10. Top them with sour cream, salsa, cheese and cilantro and enjoy

ZUCCHINI RICE NOODLES

COOKING TIME: 8 MIN | SERVES 2

INGREDIENTS:

- 1 tbsp. garlic infused oil
- 1 tbsp. ginger, grated
- 1 red chili, diced
- 1 red pepper, julienned
- 2 tbsp. fresh chives, chopped
- 1 2/3 oz. baby corn, sliced
- 1 large handful of beansprouts

- 10 ½ oz. vermicelli rice noodles
- 1 medium carrot, julienned
- 1 medium courgette, julienned
- 1 large handful spring greens, shredded
- 4 tsp. curry powder
- 1/2 tbsp. maple syrup
- 3 tbsp. tamari

- Juice of 1 lime
- 2 lime wedges (to garnish)
- 2 tbsp. fresh chopped coriander (to garnish)

DIRECTIONS:

1. Sauté garlic with oil in the Ninja Foodi's insert on SEAR/SAUTE mode for 1 minute.
2. Stir in chilly and ginger then sauté for 1 minute.
3. Add chives, baby corns and red pepper then sauté for 3 minutes.
4. Stir in a splash of water and beansprouts then cook for 2 minutes.
5. Add maple syrup, curry powder, courgette, carrots, noodles, lime juice, tamari and spring greens.
6. Mix and cook for 1 minute then garnish with lime wedges and coriander.
7. Enjoy.

PARMESAN SPAGHETTI

COOK TIME: 50 MINS | SERVES 4

INGREDIENTS:

- 1 (1-lb.) package spaghetti noodles, broken
- 3 tbsp. olive oil
- 1 tsp. salt
- 2 cups Parmesan cheese, grated
- Black pepper, to taste

DIRECTIONS:

1. Add 2 tbsp oil, 2 ½ cups water, and spaghetti to the Ninja Foodi's insert.
2. Put on the Pressure Lid and turn the pressure handle to the SEAL position.
3. Select Pressure Cook mode set the pressure to High and cooking time to 0 minutes. Hit the START/STOP button to initiate cooking.
4. Once it's done, release the pressure quickly, then remove the lid.
5. Add remaining oil, ½ cup water, cheese, black pepper, and salt to the spaghetti. Mix well and serve warm.

SPINACH ORZO

COOKING TIME: 4 MIN | SERVES 3

INGREDIENTS:

- 10 ½ oz. orzo
- 19 ¼ oz. hot vegetable stock
- 2 garlic cloves, chopped
- 3 ½ oz. fresh baby spinach
- 3 ½ oz. parmesan, grated

DIRECTIONS:

1. Add garlic, stock, and orzo to the Ninja Foodi's insert.
2. Put on the Pressure Lid and turn the pressure handle to the SEAL position.
3. Select Pressure Cook mode set the pressure to High and cooking time to 4 minutes. Hit the START/STOP button to initiate cooking.
4. Once it's done, release the pressure naturally, then remove the lid.
5. Add parmesan and spinach, then mix and leave it for 5 minutes. Serve warm.

CREAMY BUTTERNUT GNOCCHI

COOKING TIME: 10 MIN | SERVES 5

INGREDIENTS:

- 3 tsp. peanut oil
- 1 onion, sliced
- 2 garlic cloves, minced
- 1.66 lbs. butternut, seeded and diced
- 2 ½ cups gnocchi
- 1/2 tsp. salt
- 1/4 tsp. black pepper
- 10 oz. water
- 3 ½ cups heavy cream
- 2 cups fresh spinach
- juice of 1 lemon

DIRECTIONS:

1. Preheat the Ninja Foodi's insert on SEAR/SAUTE mode at High for 3 minutes.
2. Stir in garlic, onions, oil and butternut, then sauté for 4 minutes.
3. Add water, black pepper, salt and gnocchi.
4. Put on the Pressure Lid and turn the pressure handle to the SEAL position.
5. Select Pressure Cook mode set the pressure to High and cooking time to 3 minutes. Hit the START/STOP button to initiate cooking.
6. Once it's done, release the pressure naturally for 5 minutes then do a quick release, then remove the lid.
7. Add spinach, cream and lemon juice. Mix well and serve warm.

SOUPS & STEWS

CHICKEN EGG NOODLE SOUP

COOKING TIME: 27 MIN | SERVES 6

INGREDIENTS:

- 3½-lbs. whole chicken, cut in half and rinsed
- 1 yellow onion, quartered
- 1 carrot, cut into quarters
- 1 celery stalk, cut into quarters
- 2 sprigs fresh thyme
- 1 sprig fresh rosemary
- 2 fresh bay leaves
- 10 whole peppercorns

DIRECTIONS:

1. Place the chicken, carrots, thyme, and celery in the Ninja Foodi's crisping basket and set this basket inside the Ninja Foodi's insert.
2. Pour enough water to fill the Ninja Foodi's insert up to its fill line and add bay leaves, peppercorns and rosemary.
3. Put on the Pressure Lid and turn the pressure handle to the SEAL position.
4. Select Pressure Cook mode set the pressure to High and cooking time to 30 minutes. Hit the START/STOP button to initiate cooking.
5. Once it's done, release the pressure naturally, then remove the lid.
6. Empty the pot, keep the chicken aside, strain the chicken stock and discard the spices and veggies.
7. Shred the chicken and reserve it for other recipes.
8. Allow the stock to cool, pour it into a container and cover to store in the refrigerator.
9. Serve.

TEXAS BEEF CHILI

COOKING TIME: 55 MIN | SERVES 6

INGREDIENTS:

- 3 tbsp. olive oil
- 2½ lbs. boneless beef chuck, cubed
- 1 yellow onion, diced
- 2 jalapeños, seeded and diced
- 2 garlic cloves, minced
- 3 tbsp. chili powder
- 1 tbsp. cumin (ground)
- 4 cups beef broth
- 1 tbsp. salt
- 2 tbsp. masa Harina
- 1 (7.7-oz.) can chipotle salsa
- 1 (28-oz.) can crushed tomatoes
- Sour cream (to garnish)
- Grated cheese (to garnish)
- Sliced scallions (to garnish)
- Diced raw white onion (to garnish)
- Sliced jalapeños (to garnish)

DIRECTIONS:

1. Preheat oil in the Ninja Foodi's insert on SEAR/SAUTE mode at high for 6 minutes.
2. Add beef and sauté for 6 minutes.
3. Stir in cumin, chili powder, garlic, jalapenos, and onion, then sauté for 3 minutes.
4. Add broth and mix well with the beef.
5. Put on the Pressure Lid and turn the pressure handle to the SEAL position.
6. Select Pressure Cook mode set the pressure to High and cooking time to 30 minutes. Hit the START/STOP button to initiate cooking.
7. Once it's done, release the pressure quickly, then remove the lid.
8. Mix masa Harina, ¼ cup water, and salt in a bowl.
9. Add this paste along with crushed tomatoes and salsa to the Ninja Foodi's insert.
10. Switch the Ninja foodi to SEAR/SAUTE mode, then cook for 10 minutes.
11. Garnish with cream, cheese, scallions, onion, and jalapenos. Serve warm.

TORTILLA SOUP

COOKING TIME: 13 MIN | SERVES 6

INGREDIENTS:

- 3 tbsp. vegetable oil
- 1 yellow onion, diced
- 2 garlic cloves, minced
- 2 tsp. chili powder
- 2 tsp. cumin powder
- 1 tsp. coriander powder
- ½ tsp. cayenne powder

- ¼ tsp. salt
- ½ tsp. black pepper
- 4 cups vegetable broth
- 1 can chopped tomatoes, with juice
- 1 tbsp. tomato paste
- 2 cups frozen corn
- 1 can black beans, drained

- 1 bag tortilla chips
- Sliced jalapeños (to garnish)
- Diced avocado (to garnish)
- Sour cream (to garnish)
- Grated cheese (to garnish)

DIRECTIONS:

1. Sauté onion and garlic with oil in the Ninja Foodi's insert on SEAR/SAUTE mode at HI for 3 minutes.
2. Stir in cumin, chili powder, cayenne, salt, pepper and coriander, then sauté for 1 minute.
3. Add corn, tomatoes, and tomato paste, then mix gently.
4. Put on the Pressure Lid and turn the pressure handle to the SEAL position.
5. Select Pressure Cook mode set the pressure to High and cooking time to 0 minutes. Hit the START/STOP button to initiate cooking.
6. Once it's done, release the pressure quickly, then remove the lid.
7. Serve warm with tortilla chips, jalapenos, avocado, sour cream, and cheese on top

CHICKEN MUSHROOM RAMEN

COOKING TIME: 35 MIN | SERVES 6

INGREDIENTS:

- 1 (4-lb.) chicken, giblets removed
- 2-inch ginger, chopped
- 1 yellow onion, halved
- 5 garlic cloves, minced
- 6 dried shiitake mushrooms

- ¼ cup Dijon mustard
- 1 tbsp. salt
- 2 tsp. soy sauce
- 6 portions Instant ramen noodles
- Lemon zest (to garnish)

DIRECTIONS:

1. Stuff the chicken with onion, garlic, and ginger, then place it in the Ninja Foodi's crisping basket.
2. Set the basket inside the Ninja Foodi's insert and add mushrooms around the chicken.
3. Pour 6 cups of water into the Ninja Foodi's insert.
4. Put on the Pressure Lid and turn the pressure handle to the SEAL position.
5. Select Pressure Cook mode set the pressure to High and cooking time to 30 minutes. Hit the START/STOP button to initiate cooking.
6. Once it's done, release the pressure naturally, then remove the lid.
7. Strain the broth into the bowl and keep the mushrooms caps.
8. Transfer the chicken to the cutting board and shred its meat while removing the cartilage and bones.
9. Reserve half of the shredded chicken in a bowl and refrigerate for later use.
10. Return the remaining half of the chicken, broth, and mushrooms to the Ninja Foodi's insert.
11. Switch the Ninja food to SEAR/SAUTE mode on High and cook for 5 minutes.
12. Stir in soy sauce, salt and mustard, then mix well.
13. Divide the noodles into 6 bowls and pour the broth over them.
14. Add mushrooms, shredded chicken, and lemon zest on top. Serve warm.

VEGAN BEAN CHILI

COOKING TIME: 66 MIN | SERVES 6

INGREDIENTS:

- 1 lb. dried kidney beans
- 2 tsp. 1 tbsp. salt
- 3 tbsp. olive oil
- 1 lb. button mushrooms caps, quartered
- 2 cups raw pecans, chopped
- 2 jalapeños, halved, seeded, and diced
- 1 yellow onion, finely diced

- 1 bell pepper, green, seeded and diced
- 1 tbsp. chili powder
- 1 tbsp. cumin (ground)
- 1 tbsp. dried oregano
- 1 cinnamon stick
- 1 (28-oz.) can diced tomatoes
- 2 cups vegetable broth

- 1 (15-oz.) can tomato sauce
- Grated dairy-free cheese (to garnish)

DIRECTIONS:

1. Spread beans in the Ninja Crisping Basket and insert it in the Ninja Foodi's insert.
2. Add 6 cups water and 2 tsp salt to the Ninja Foodi's insert.
3. Put on the Pressure Lid and turn the pressure handle to the SEAL position.
4. Select Pressure Cook mode set the pressure to High and cooking time to 30 minutes. Hit the START/STOP button to initiate cooking.
5. Once it's done, release the pressure naturally, then remove the lid.
6. Remove the beans and transfer to a bowl.
7. Empty the Ninja Foodi's insert and switch the Ninja foodi to the SEAR/SAUTE mode at high.
8. Stir in oil and mushrooms, then sauté for 6 minutes.
9. Add cinnamon stick, beans, tomato sauce, 1 tbsp salt, broth, tomatoes, oregano, cumin, chili powder, bell pepper, onion, jalapenos, and pecans.
10. Cook for 30 minutes on SEAR/SAUTE mode at medium heat.
11. Garnish with cheese and serve warm.

TOMATO CARROT SOUP

COOK TIME: 50 MINS | SERVES 4

INGREDIENTS:

- 3 carrots, chopped
- 1 onion, diced
- 1 tbsp. olive oil
- 2 garlic cloves, minced
- 1 (28 oz.) can crush tomatoes
- 1 tbsp. tomato paste
- 1 cup vegetable broth

- ¼ tsp. dried oregano
- ¼ cup basil, chopped
- Salt and black pepper, to taste

DIRECTIONS:

1. Preheat oil in the Ninja Foodi's insert on SEAR/SAUTE mode for 5 minutes.
2. Stir in garlic, then sauté for 30 seconds.
3. Add vegetable broth and rest of the ingredients, then mix well.
4. Put on the Pressure Lid and turn the pressure handle to the SEAL position.
5. Select Pressure Cook mode set the pressure to High and cooking time to 15 minutes. Hit the START/STOP button to initiate cooking.
6. Once it's done, release the pressure naturally, then remove the lid.
7. Puree the tomato carrot soup with a hand blender until smooth.
8. Serve warm.

HERBED CHICKEN STOCK

COOKING TIME: 30 MIN | SERVES 8

INGREDIENTS:

- 3½-lbs. whole chicken, cut in half and rinsed
- 1 yellow onion, quartered
- 1 carrot, cut into quarters
- 1 celery stalk, cut into quarters
- 2 sprigs fresh thyme
- 1 sprig fresh rosemary
- 2 fresh bay leaves
- 10 whole peppercorns

DIRECTIONS:

1. Place the chicken, carrots, thyme, and celery in the Ninja Foodi's crisping basket and set this basket inside the Ninja Foodi's insert.
2. Pour enough water to fill the Ninja Foodi's insert up to its fill line and add bay leaves, peppercorns and rosemary.
3. Put on the Pressure Lid and turn the pressure handle to the SEAL position.
4. Select Pressure Cook mode set the pressure to High and cooking time to 30 minutes. Hit the START/STOP button to initiate cooking.
5. Once it's done, release the pressure naturally, then remove the lid.
6. Empty the pot, keep the chicken aside, strain the chicken stock and discard the spices and veggies.
7. Shred the chicken and reserve it for other recipes.
8. Allow the stock to cool, pour it into a container and cover to store in the refrigerator.
9. Serve.

SHRIMP SAUSAGE GUMBO

COOKING TIME: 81 MIN | SERVES 6

INGREDIENTS:

- 14 oz. andouille sausage, cut into rounds
- ¼ cup 2 tbsp. all-purpose flour
- 2 tbsp. olive oil
- 2 celery stalks, diced
- 1 green bell pepper, seeded and diced
- 1 yellow onion, diced
- 4 garlic cloves, minced
- 24 frozen shrimp, peeled, and deveined
- 3 cups seafood stock
- 2 sprigs fresh thyme
- 2 dried bay leaves
- 1 tbsp. salt
- ½ tsp. black pepper
- ½ tsp. cayenne

DIRECTIONS:

1. Place the sausage in the Ninja Crisping Basket and insert it into the Ninja Foodi's insert.
2. Put on the crisping lid and cook on AIR CRISP mode for 20 minutes at 390 °F.
3. Transfer the crispy cooked sausage to a bowl and leave its fat in the Ninja Foodi's insert.
4. Stir in ¼ cup flour and oil, then put on the crisping lid and cook on AIR CRIPS mode at 390 °F for 45 minutes.
5. Switch the ninja foodi to SEAR/SAUTE mode.
6. Toss in bell pepper, celery, onion, and garlic, then sauté for 10 minutes.
7. Add shrimp, thyme, bay leaves, cayenne, salt, 2 tbsp stock, and black pepper.
8. Put on the Pressure Lid and turn the pressure handle to the SEAL position.
9. Select Pressure Cook mode set the pressure to High and cooking time to 1 minute. Hit the START/STOP button to initiate cooking.
10. Once it's done, release the pressure quickly, then remove the lid.
11. Mix flour with 2 tbsp stock in a bowl and pour into the Ninja Foodi's insert.
12. Cook for 5 minutes on SEAR/SAUTE mode until the soup thickens.
13. Garnish with thyme and serve warm.

BEEF PHO

COOKING TIME: 84 MIN | SERVES 6

INGREDIENTS:

- 2 tbsp. olive oil
- 2½ lbs. eye of round beef
- 5 whole cloves
- 4 green cardamom pods
- 2-star anise pods
- 2 tsp. coriander seeds
- 1 tsp. whole black peppercorns

- 1 cinnamon stick
- ½ yellow onion
- 2 carrots, halved
- 1 (3-inch) piece ginger, halved
- Cooking spray
- 2½ lbs. beef soup bones
- 3 tbsp. fish sauce

- 2 tbsp. light brown sugar
- 1 tbsp. salt
- 8 oz. thin rice noodles
- Lime wedges (to garnish)
- Fresh jalapeño slices (to garnish)
- Thai basil leaves (to garnish)

DIRECTIONS:

1. Preheat olive oil in the Ninja Foodi's insert on SEAR/SAUTE mode at High for 6 minutes.
2. Add beef to the Ninja Foodi's insert and sear it for 4 minutes per side.
3. Stir in cloves, star anise, coriander, cinnamon stick, peppercorns, and cardamom. Sauté for 1 minute.
4. Push the beef to a side and set the reversible rack in the Ninja Foodi's insert.
5. Add ginger, carrots, and onion to the rack and spray with cooking oil.
6. Put on the crisping lid and cook on BROIL mode for 12 minutes.
7. Remove the reversible rack and transfer the veggies to the beef.
8. Add beef soup and water to fill the pot. Put on the Pressure Lid and turn the pressure handle to the SEAL position.
9. Select Pressure Cook mode set the pressure to High and cooking time to 45 minutes. Hit the START/STOP button to initiate cooking.
10. Once it's done, release the pressure quickly, then remove the lid.
11. Remove the meat from the Ninja Foodi's insert and wrap the beef in a plastic wrap.
12. Discard the veggies and bones from the pot.
13. Add brown sugar, fish sauce, and salt to the Ninja Foodi's insert.
14. Mix well and then pour into a bowl. Allow the broth to cool, then skim off the fats.
15. Pour 16 cups of water into the Ninja Foodi's insert and cook for 15 minutes on SEAR/SAUTE mode.
16. Add noodles to the Ninja Crisping Basket and place it in the Ninja Foodi's insert.
17. Cook for 6 minutes on SEAR/SAUTE mode.
18. Divide the noodles into the serving bowls.
19. Empty the Ninja Foodi's insert and pour the broth into the pot, then cook for 10 minutes on SEAR/SAUTE mode.
20. Unwrap the beef and slice it. Divide the broth into the serving bowl and add the slices of beef.
21. Garnish and enjoy.

CHICKEN PASTA SOUP

COOKING TIME: 0 MIN | SERVES 6

INGREDIENTS:

- 8 cups chicken stock
- 2 cups cooked chicken meat, shredded
- 1 carrot, chopped

- 1 celery stalk, chopped
- 12 oz. dried rotini pasta
- 1 tbsp. parsley, minced

- Salt, to taste

DIRECTIONS:

1. Add shredded chicken, stock, carrot, pasta, celery, and carrot to the Ninja Foodi's insert.
2. Put on the Pressure Lid and turn the pressure handle to the SEAL position.
3. Select Pressure Cook mode set the pressure to High and cooking time to 0 minutes. Hit the START/STOP button to initiate cooking.
4. Once it's done, release the pressure naturally, then remove the lid.
5. Add salt and parsley.
6. Serve warm.

MUSHROOM BARLEY SOUP

COOKING TIME: 23 MIN | SERVES 6

INGREDIENTS:

- 3 tbsp. olive oil
- 1 lb. baby portobello
- 2 cups pearled barley
- 1 yellow onion, diced
- 3 sprigs fresh thyme
- 8 cups beef broth
- 2 tbsp. Worcestershire sauce
- 2 tsp. salt
- ½ tsp. black pepper

DIRECTIONS:

1. Mix mushrooms with oil in the Ninja Foodi's insert and put on the crisping lid.
2. Cook on AIR CRISP mode for 5 minutes at 390 °F.
3. Switch the Ninja Foodi to SEAR/SAUTE mode at high.
4. Stir in barley and sauté for 8 minutes.
5. Add broth, thyme, and onion.
6. Put on the Pressure Lid and turn the pressure handle to the SEAL position.
7. Select Pressure Cook mode set the pressure to High and cooking time to 18 minutes. Hit the START/STOP button to initiate cooking.
8. Once it's done, release the pressure naturally, then remove the lid.
9. Add black pepper, salt, and Worcestershire sauce.
10. Serve warm.

BEEF MUSHROOM STEW

COOKING TIME: 45 MIN | SERVES 6

INGREDIENTS:

- 4 lbs. boneless beef stew, cubed
- 8 oz. fresh shiitake mushrooms
- 4 celery stalks, quartered
- 4 garlic cloves, smashed
- 3 medium carrots, quartered
- 1 yellow onion, quartered
- 1½ lbs. new red potatoes, quartered
- 3 fresh sage leaves
- 2 dried bay leaves
- 2 sprigs fresh thyme
- 10 black peppercorn
- 4 cups beef broth
- 2 tbsp. Worcestershire sauce
- 2 tbsp. tomato paste
- 2 tbsp. soy sauce
- 1 tbsp. maple syrup
- 1 tbsp. Dijon mustard
- ¼ cup flour
- Salt, to taste to taste
- Fresh thyme (to garnish)
- Cracked black pepper (to garnish)

DIRECTIONS:

1. Add beef, garlic, celery, mushrooms, sage, potatoes, onion, carrots, thyme, bay leaves, soy sauce, maple syrup, Dijon mustard, tomato paste, 3 ½ cups broth, Worcestershire sauce, and peppercorns to the Ninja Foodi's insert.
2. Put on the Pressure Lid and turn the pressure handle to the SEAL position.
3. Select Pressure Cook mode set the pressure to High and cooking time to 40 minutes. Hit the START/STOP button to initiate cooking.
4. Once it's done, release the pressure quickly, then remove the lid.
5. Mix ½ cup broth with flour in a small bowl.
6. Pour this slurry into the stew and cook on SEAR/SAUTE mode for 5 minutes until it thickens.
7. Discard the bay leaves and add salt for seasoning.
8. Garnish with black pepper and thyme.
9. Serve warm.

CLAM POTATO CHOWDER

COOKING TIME: 40 MIN | SERVES 6

INGREDIENTS:

- 3 tbsp. olive oil
- 2 carrots, diced
- 2 celery stalks, diced
- 1 yellow onion, diced
- 2 garlic cloves, minced
- 6 strips bacon, chopped
- 2 (6.5-oz.) cans chopped clams, with juice
- 1 lb. fresh clams, rinsed and scrubbed
- 2 russet potatoes, peeled and diced
- 2 cups heavy cream
- 1½ cups whole milk
- ½ cup clam juice
- 2 sprigs fresh thyme
- 1 tsp. salt
- Chopped fresh dill (to garnish)
- Tarragon (to garnish)
- Parsley (to garnish)
- Chives (to garnish)
- Chervil (to garnish)
- Oyster crackers (to garnish)

DIRECTIONS:

1. Preheat oil in Ninja Foodi's insert on SEAR/SAUTE mode at High for 5 minutes.
2. Stir in garlic, onion, celery, and carrots, then sauté for 6 minutes.
3. Add bacon, then sauté for 12 minutes until crispy.
4. Stir in clams, juices, and potatoes and mix gently.
5. Put on the Pressure Lid and turn the pressure handle to the SEAL position.
6. Select Pressure Cook mode set the pressure to High and cooking time to 2 minutes. Hit the START/STOP button to initiate cooking.
7. Once it's done, release the pressure quickly, then remove the lid.
8. Stir in thyme sprigs, cream, milk, and salt, then switch the Ninja Foodi to SEAR/SAUTE mode at medium heat.
9. Cook for 15 minutes, then garnish with dill, tarragon, parsley, chives, chervil, and oyster crackers.
10. Serve warm.

BUTTERNUT SQUASH SOUP

COOKING TIME: 64 MIN | SERVES 6

INGREDIENTS:

- 4 cups balsamic vinegar
- 4 tbsp. unsalted butter
- 1 yellow onion, diced
- 2 garlic cloves, minced
- 8 fresh sage leaves
- 1 (2-lbs.) butternut, peeled, and cubed
- 1 Golden apple, peeled, cored, and cubes
- 4 cups vegetable broth
- 2 tsp. salt
- Crumbled blue cheese (to garnish)

DIRECTIONS:

1. Add vinegar to Ninja Foodi's insert and cook on SEAR/SAUTE mode at High for 30 minutes.
2. Transfer the reduced vinegar to a bowl and allow it to cool.
3. Add butter to the Ninja Foodi's insert and melt it for 8 minutes.
4. Stir in sage, garlic, and onion, then sauté for 7 minutes.
5. Add broth, apple, and squash and mix gently.
6. Put on the Pressure Lid and turn the pressure handle to the SEAL position.
7. Select Pressure Cook mode set the pressure to High and cooking time to 10 minutes. Hit the START/STOP button to initiate cooking.
8. Once it's done, release the pressure quickly, then remove the lid.
9. Add salt and lightly mash the squash mixture with a potato masher.
10. Switch the Ninja foodi to the SEAR/SAUTE mode and cook for 10 minutes.
11. Garnish with cheese and balsamic vinegar.
12. Serve warm.

CREAMY CHEESE SOUP

COOKING TIME: 14 MIN | SERVES 6

INGREDIENTS:

- 3 tbsp. olive oil
- 1 yellow onion, diced
- 3 garlic cloves, minced
- 5 allspice berries
- 2 dried bay leaves
- ½ tsp. turmeric (ground)
- 2 tbsp. Dijon mustard
- 4 (12-oz.) bottles of lager
- 16 oz. sharp cheddar cheese, shredded
- ¼ cup flour
- 1 cup heavy cream
- 3 tbsp. sugar
- 1 tbsp. salt

DIRECTIONS:

1. Preheat oil in the Ninja Foodi's insert on SEAR/SAUTE mode at High for 5 minutes.
2. Stir in bay leaves, allspice, garlic, and onion, then sauté for 4 minutes.
3. Stir in mustard and turmeric, then sauté for 2 minutes and pour in the beer.
4. Put on the Pressure Lid and turn the pressure handle to the SEAL position.
5. Select Pressure Cook mode set the pressure to High and cooking time to 0 minutes. Hit the START/STOP button to initiate cooking.
6. Once it's done, release the pressure quickly, then remove the lid.
7. Mix cheese with flour in a bowl, then add to the Ninja Foodi's insert.
8. Switch the Ninja Foodi to SEAR/SAUTE mode at High and cook for 3 minutes.
9. Stir in salt, sugar, and cream, then mix well.
10. Discard the bay leaves and serve warm.

CHEESY BROCCOLI SOUP

COOKING TIME: 31 MIN | SERVES 6

INGREDIENTS:

- 4 cups broccoli florets
- Cooking spray
- 3 tbsp. olive oil
- 1 yellow onion, diced
- 3 garlic cloves, minced
- 2 dried bay leaves
- 2 tbsp. Dijon mustard
- 8 cups vegetable broth
- 16 oz. cheddar cheese, shredded
- ¼ cup flour
- 1 cup heavy cream
- 2 tsp. salt

DIRECTIONS:

1. Spread half of the broccoli florets in the Ninja Crisping Basket and insert it in the Ninja Foodi's insert.
2. Spray them with cooking spray and put on the crisping lid.
3. Cook on AIR CRISP mode for 12 minutes at 390 °F.
4. Transfer the broccoli to a bowl and allow it to cool, then empty the pot.
5. Chop the remaining broccoli and keep it aside.
6. Add oil to Ninja Foodi's insert and sauté on SEAR/SAUTE mode at High for 5 minutes.
7. Stir in onion, bay leaves, chopped broccoli, onion, and garlic, then sauté for 7 minutes.
8. Add broth and mustard, then mix well.
9. Put on the Pressure Lid and turn the pressure handle to the SEAL position.
10. Select Pressure Cook mode set the pressure to High and cooking time to 2 minutes. Hit the START/STOP button to initiate cooking.
11. Once it's done, release the pressure quickly, then remove the lid.
12. Mix cheese with flour in a bowl and add to the Ninja Foodi's insert.
13. Switch the Ninja Foodi to the SEAR/SAUTE mode.
14. Discard the bay leaves and cook for 2 minutes.
15. Stir in cream and salt, then cook for 3 minutes with occasional stirring.
16. Garnish with broccoli florets. Serve warm.

PORK CHILE STEW

COOKING TIME: 54 MIN | SERVES 6

INGREDIENTS:

- ¼ cup olive oil
- 2½ lbs. boneless pork shoulder, cubed
- 1 lb. frozen flame-roasted New Mexico green chiles
- 4 garlic cloves, minced
- 1 yellow onion, diced

- 1 tbsp. 2 tsp. salt
- 2 tsp. cumin (ground)
- 2 tsp. dried oregano
- 4 cups chicken stock
- 2 russet potatoes, peeled and diced
- ¼ cup flour

- Fresh cilantro (to garnish)
- Sour cream (to garnish)
- Grated cheese (to garnish)
- Sliced scallions (to garnish)

DIRECTIONS:

1. Preheat oil in the Ninja Foodi's insert on SEAR/SAUTE mode at high for 6 minutes.
2. Add pork and sauté for 10 minutes until brown.
3. Stir in stock, oregano, cumin, salt, onion, garlic, and chiles.
4. Put on the Pressure Lid and turn the pressure handle to the SEAL position.
5. Select Pressure Cook mode set the pressure to High and cooking time to 30 minutes. Hit the START/STOP button to initiate cooking.
6. Once it's done, release the pressure quickly, then remove the lid.
7. Add potatoes to the pork mixture and mix gently.
8. Put on the Pressure Lid and turn the pressure handle to the SEAL position.
9. Select Pressure Cook mode set the pressure to High and cooking time to 3 minutes. Hit the START/STOP button to initiate cooking.
10. Once it's done, release the pressure quickly, then remove the lid.
11. Add flour and switch to the SEAR/SAUTE mode at MD: HI.
12. Cook for 5 minutes with occasional stirring.
13. Garnish with cilantro, sour cream, cheese, and scallions.
14. Serve warm.

PORK FEIJOADA

COOKING TIME: 62 MIN | SERVES 8

INGREDIENTS:

- 3 tbsp. olive oil
- 12 oz. smoked pork, cut into chunks
- 6 slices bacon, cut in half crosswise
- 2½ lbs. pork spare ribs
- 2½ lbs. boneless pork stew meat
- 10 garlic cloves, smashed

- 2 lbs. dried black beans, rinsed
- 1 tbsp. salt
- Orange slices (to garnish)

DIRECTIONS:

1. Preheat oil in the Ninja Foodi's insert on SEAR/SAUTE mode at high for 5 minutes.
2. Add bacon and sausage, then sauté for 12 minutes.
3. Transfer the sausage-bacon mixture to a bowl and leave the fats in the Ninja Foodi's insert.
4. Add ribs, stew meat, beans, garlic, and enough water to reach the fill line.
5. Put on the Pressure Lid and turn the pressure handle to the SEAL position.
6. Select Pressure Cook mode set the pressure to High and cooking time to 45 minutes. Hit the START/STOP button to initiate cooking.
7. Once it's done, release the pressure naturally, then remove the lid.
8. Add feijoada and mix well while breaking it.
9. Stir in bacon, sausage, and salt.
10. Serve warm.

CORN JALAPENO CHOWDER

COOKING TIME: 43 MIN | SERVES 4

INGREDIENTS:

- 6 ears corn, kernels and cobs separated
- Cooking spray
- 3 tbsp. corn oil
- 1 yellow onion, diced
- 1 garlic clove, minced
- 1 jalapeño, seeded and minced
- 1 chipotle chile in adobo sauce, minced
- 1 can unsweetened coconut milk
- 2 tsp. salt
- Chopped fresh cilantro (to garnish)
- Lime wedges (to garnish)
- Crumbled Cotija cheese (to garnish)

DIRECTIONS:

1. Spread half of the kernels in the Ninja Crisping Basket and spray them with cooking spray.
2. Place the Ninja Crisping Basket in the Ninja Foodi's insert and put on the crisping lid.
3. Cook on AIR CRISP mode for 17 minutes at 390 °F.
4. Remove the corn and basket from the Ninja Foodi's insert. Keep the kernels in a bowl.
5. Preheat our in the Ninja Foodi's insert on SEAR/SAUTE mode at High for 5 minutes.
6. Stir in chipotle chile, jalapeno, garlic, and onion, then sauté for 6 minutes.
7. Add remaining corn kernels, corn cobs, and enough water to reach the 10-cup line.
8. Put on the Pressure Lid and turn the pressure handle to the SEAL position.
9. Select Pressure Cook mode set the pressure to High and cooking time to 10 minutes. Hit the START/STOP button to initiate cooking.
10. Once it's done, release the pressure quickly, then remove the lid.
11. Remove and discard the corn cobs, then puree the chowder using an immersion blender.
12. Add salt, crispy corn, and coconut milk, then switch the Ninja Foodi to SEAR/SAUTE mode at high.
13. Cook for 5 minutes with occasional stirring.
14. Garnish with cilantro, lime wedges, and cheese. Serve warm.

POTATO CREAM SOUP

COOKING TIME: 19 MIN | SERVES 4

INGREDIENTS:

- 1 large onion, chopped
- 2 tbsp. butter
- 1 tsp. thyme leaves
- 2 garlic cloves, minced
- 4 cups chicken broth
- 6 russet potatoes, peeled and diced
- 1 cup 2 tbsp. milk
- 2 tbsp. cornstarch
- ½ cup heavy cream
- Salt and black pepper, to taste
- Cheddar cheese, shredded

DIRECTIONS:

1. Melt butter in the Ninja Foodi's insert on SEAR/SAUTE mode for 5 minutes.
2. Stir in garlic and thyme, then sauté for 1 minute.
3. Add potatoes, salt, black pepper, and broth mix well.
4. Put on the Pressure Lid and turn the pressure handle to the SEAL position.
5. Select Pressure Cook mode set the pressure to High and cooking time to 8 minutes. Hit the START/STOP button to initiate cooking.
6. Once it's done, release the pressure quickly, then remove the lid.
7. Mix cornstarch with 2 tbsp milk in a bowl and pour into the Ninja Foodi's insert.
8. Switch the Ninja foodi to SEAR/SAUTE mode.
9. Add cream, slurry, and remaining milk to the Ninja Foodi's insert and cook for 5 minutes with occasional stirring.
10. Garnish with cheese and serve warm.

CHEESEBURGER SOUP

COOKING TIME: 20 MIN | SERVES 8

INGREDIENTS:

- 1 lb ground beef
- 1/2 tsp salt
- Black pepper, to taste
- 2 sweet onions, diced
- 5 baby Yukon gold potatoes, cubed
- 3 carrots, sliced
- 4 garlic cloves, minced
- 2 tbsp parsley, chopped
- 1 tbsp mustard (ground)
- 1/2 tsp dill weed
- 2 cups chicken broth
- 1 cup yogurt
- 1/2 cup cheddar powder

DIRECTIONS:

1. Sauté beef with black pepper, salt, and cooking spray in the Ninja Foodi's insert on SEAR/SAUTE mode for 5 minutes.
2. Stir in garlic, onion, carrots, broth, dill weed, mustard, parsley, and potatoes.
3. Put on the Pressure Lid and turn the pressure handle to the SEAL position.
4. Select Pressure Cook mode set the pressure to High and cooking time to 10 minutes. Hit the START/STOP button to initiate cooking.
5. Once it's done, release the pressure quickly, then remove the lid.
6. Stir in yogurt, and cheddar cheese, then switch the Ninja Foodi to the SEAR/SAUTE mode.
7. Cook for 5 minutes with occasional stirring.
8. Serve warm.

ITALIAN MEATBALL SOUP

COOKING TIME: 28 MIN | SERVES 8

INGREDIENTS:

Meatballs
- 1½ lbs. 80% lean ground beef
- 12 oz. ground pork
- 1 cup Italian-flavored breadcrumbs
- ¼ cup milk
- ¼ cup Parmesan cheese, shredded
- 1 large egg, beaten

- 8 fresh basil leaves, chopped
- 4 garlic cloves, minced
- 2½ tsp. salt
- 1 tsp. red pepper flakes
- Cooking spray

Soup
- 3 fresh basil leaves

- 2 garlic cloves, smashed
- 1 tsp. fennel seeds
- 8 cups chicken stock
- 1 large egg, beaten
- ¼ cup Parmesan cheese, grated
- 2 tsp. salt
- 2 cups trimmed fresh spinach

DIRECTIONS:

1. Mix all the ingredients for the pork-beef meatballs in a bowl and make 8 meatballs out of it.
2. Place these meatballs in the Ninja Crisping Basket and insert it into the Ninja Foodi's insert. Spray them with cooking spray.
3. Put on the crisping lid and cook on BROIL mode for 20 minutes.
4. Transfer the meatballs to a plate and remove the basket from the Ninja Foodi's insert.
5. Switch the ninja foodi to the SEAR/SAUTE mode.
6. Stir in fennel seeds, garlic, and basil leaves and sauté for 4 minutes.
7. Return the meatballs to the pot and pour in the stock.
8. Put on the Pressure Lid and turn the pressure handle to the SEAL position.
9. Select Pressure Cook mode set the pressure to High and cooking time to 1 minute. Hit the START/STOP button to initiate cooking.
10. Once it's done, release the pressure quickly, then remove the lid.
11. Switch the Ninja foodi to SEAR/SAUTE mode.
12. Mix cheese and egg in a bowl and pour into the Ninja Foodi's insert.
13. Add this cheese mixture, spinach, and salt to the soup and cook for 3 minutes with occasional stirring.
14. Garnish with red pepper flakes and serve warm.

PARMESAN LENTIL SOUP

COOKING TIME: 21 MIN | SERVES 4

INGREDIENTS:

- 2 stalks celery, chopped
- 1 large onion, chopped
- 1 carrot, peeled and chopped
- 3 garlic cloves, minced
- 2 tsp. thyme
- 1 ½ cup green lentils
- 1 can diced tomatoes

- 1 tsp. Italian seasoning
- 4 cup chicken broth
- 4 cup baby spinach
- Salt and black pepper, to taste
- Parmesan, grated

DIRECTIONS:

1. Add onion, celery, carrot, tomatoes, garlic, lentils, thyme, seasoning, and broth to the Ninja Foodi's insert.
2. Put on the Pressure Lid and turn the pressure handle to the SEAL position.
3. Select Pressure Cook mode, set the pressure to High and cooking time to 18 minutes. Hit the START/STOP button to initiate cooking.
4. Once it's done, release the pressure quickly, then remove the lid.
5. Stir in spinach and parmesan then mix gently.
6. Serve after 3 minutes.
7. Enjoy.

AU GRATIN SOUP

COOKING TIME: 35MIN | SERVES 4

INGREDIENTS:

- 2 tbsp. butter
- 1 tbsp. soy sauce
- 2 onions, peeled and chopped
- 1 tbsp. tomato paste
- 32 oz. beef stock
- 1 tbsp. Worcestershire sauce
- 4 cups crusty French bread, cut into cubes

- 2 cups Mozzarella cheese, shredded
- 1 tsp. salt
- Black pepper, to taste

DIRECTIONS:

1. Melt butter in the Ninja Foodi's insert on SEAR/SAUTE mode for 5 minutes.
2. Stir in onions, then sauté for 10 minutes.
3. Add black pepper, salt, Worcestershire sauce, tomato sauce, and soy sauce and cook for 5 minutes.
4. Stir in beef stock and cook for another 5 minutes.
5. Put on the Pressure Lid and turn the pressure handle to the SEAL position.
6. Select Pressure Cook mode set the pressure to High and cooking time to 15 minutes. Hit the START/STOP button to initiate cooking.
7. Once it's done, release the pressure quickly, then remove the lid.
8. Add bread cubes and cheese on top of this soup
9. Switch the Ninja foodi to BROIL mode, cover with crisping lid and cook for 8 minutes.
10. Serve warm.

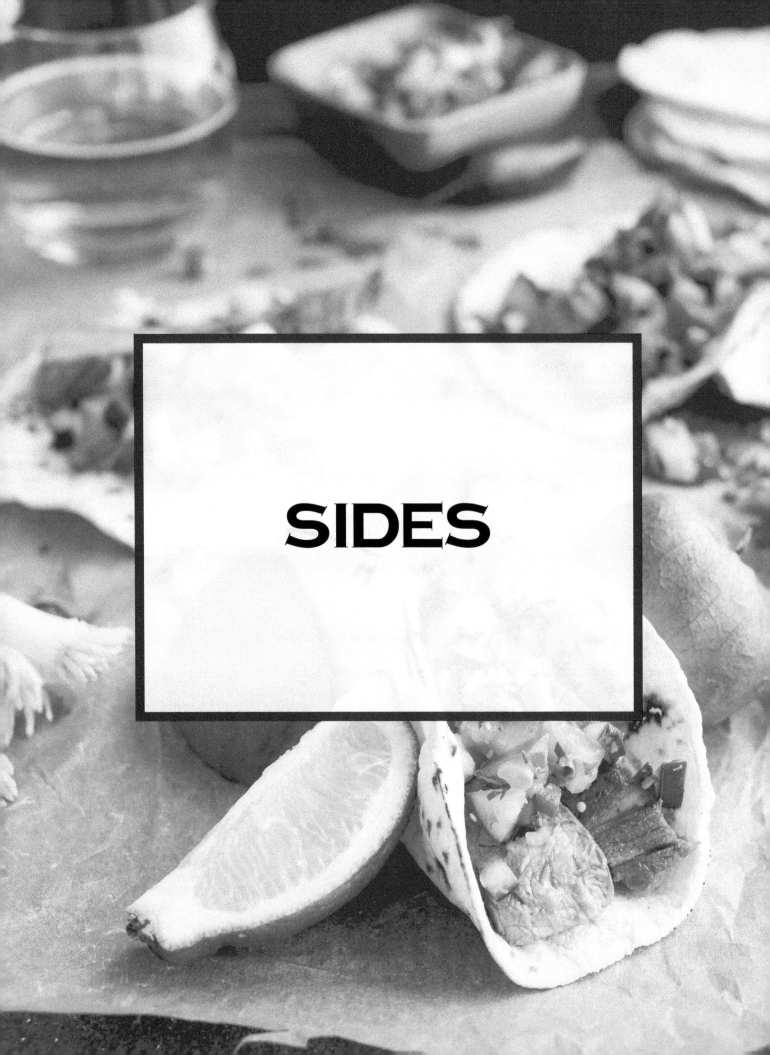

SIDES

CREAMY BACON MASHED POTATOES

COOKING TIME: 8 MIN | SERVES 8

INGREDIENTS:

- 3 lbs. potatoes, peeled and quartered
- 1 ½ cups chicken broth
- 1 ½ tsp. salt
- 4 tsp. butter, salted
- ¼ cup sour cream
- ¼ cup milk
- ½ tsp. black pepper
- ½ cup cheddar cheese, shredded
- ¼ cup bacon, cooked
- ¼ cup green onions, sliced

DIRECTIONS:

1. Add potato quarters, salt and chicken broth to the Ninja Foodi's insert.
2. Put on the Pressure Lid and turn the pressure handle to the SEAL position.
3. Select Pressure Cook mode, set the pressure to High and cooking time to 8 minutes. Hit the START/STOP button to initiate cooking.
4. Once it's done, release the pressure naturally, then remove the lid.
5. Remove the cooking liquid from the pot leaving only ½ of cup of liquid.
6. Mash the potatoes with a potato masher then add butter, black pepper, ½ tsp. salt, milk and sour cream.
7. Mix well then stir in bacon and cheese.
8. Mix again, then garnish with green onions.
9. Serve warm.

PARMESAN BROCCOLI FLORETS

COOKING TIME: 8 MIN | SERVES 4

INGREDIENTS:

- 12 oz. fresh broccoli florets
- 1 tsp. vegetable oil
- ¼ tsp. salt
- 1 pinch of black pepper
- ½ cup Parmesan cheese, shredded

DIRECTIONS:

1. Spread the broccoli florets in the Ninja crisping basket and insert it into the Ninja Foodi's insert.
2. Pour ½ cup water into the Ninja Foodi's insert.
3. Put on the Pressure Lid and turn the pressure handle to the SEAL position.
4. Select Pressure Cook mode, set the pressure to High and cooking time to 0 minutes. Hit the START/STOP button to initiate cooking.
5. Once it's done, release the pressure quickly, then remove the lid.
6. Transfer the broccoli florets to a bowl.
7. Toss in parmesan, black pepper, salt and oil then mix well.
8. Return the broccoli to the Ninja crisping basket and place it back in the Ninja Foodi's insert.
9. Put on the crisping lid and cook on AIR CRISP mode at 390 degrees F for 8 minutes.
10. Garnish the broccoli with parmesan cheese.
11. Serve warm.

CHEESY CAULIFLOWER FLORETS

COOKING TIME: 10 MIN | SERVES 4

INGREDIENTS:

- 1 cauliflower head, cut into florets
- 8 2/3 oz water
- 17 ½ oz milk
- 1 2/3 oz butter, cubed
- 1 2/3 oz plain flour
- 1 tsp. dried mustard powder
- Salt and black pepper, to taste
- 3 ½ oz mature cheddar cheese, grated

DIRECTIONS:

1. Add cauliflower florets and water to the Ninja Foodi's insert.
2. Put on the Pressure Lid and turn the pressure handle to the SEAL position.
3. Select Pressure Cook mode, set the pressure to LOW and cooking time to 1 minute. Hit the START/STOP button to initiate cooking.
4. Once it's done, release the pressure quickly, then remove the lid.
5. Transfer the cauliflower to a colander and empty the pot.
6. Switch the Ninja foodi to the SEAR/SAUTE mode at MD: HI heat.
7. Add butter, milk and flour to the Ninja Foodi's insert, mix and cook for 2 minutes until it thickens.
8. Stir in mustard, half of the cheese, seasoning and cauliflower.
9. Put on the crisping lid and cook AIR CRISP mode at 390 degrees F for 7 minutes.
10. Garnish with remaining cheese and serve warm.

FRIED BLACK BEANS

COOKING TIME: 40 MIN | SERVES 6

INGREDIENTS:

- 1-lb. dried black beans, rinsed
- ½ medium yellow onion, diced
- 2 garlic cloves, minced
- 1 tsp. cumin (ground)
- 1 tsp. salt
- 2 tsp. vegetable oil

DIRECTIONS:

1. Add 4 cups water, cumin, salt, garlic, onion and beans to the Ninja Foodi's insert.
2. Put on the Pressure Lid and turn the pressure handle to the SEAL position.
3. Select Pressure Cook mode, set the pressure to High and cooking time to 30 minutes. Hit the START/STOP button to initiate cooking.
4. Once it's done, release the pressure naturally, then remove the lid.
5. Strain the beans and transfer them to a bowl along with ¼ cup cooking liquid.
6. Mash the beans with a fork until chunky.
7. Add oil and mashed beans to the Ninja Foodi's insert.
8. Switch the Ninja foodi to SEAR/SAUTE mode and sauté for 10 minutes.
9. Stir in salt, then mix well.
10. Serve warm.

HAM WITH GREENS

COOKING TIME: 12 MIN | SERVES 6

INGREDIENTS:

- 2 tsp. butter, unsalted
- 1 yellow onion, diced
- 2 garlic cloves, minced
- 1 smoked ham hock
- 2 cups chicken stock
- 2 lbs. collard greens, sliced
- Juice of 1 lemon
- 2 tsp. salt

DIRECTIONS:

1. Melt butter in the Ninja Foodi's insert on SEAR/SAUTE mode at High for 4 minutes.
2. Stir in garlic and onion, then sauté for 5 minutes.
3. Add the stock, ham hock and collard greens.
4. Put on the Pressure Lid and turn the pressure handle to the SEAL position.
5. Select Pressure Cook mode, set the pressure to High and cooking time to 3 minutes. Hit the START/STOP button to initiate cooking.
6. Once it's done, release the pressure quickly, then remove the lid.
7. Stir in salt, and lemon juice, then mix well.
8. Serve warm.

CHEESY POTATO JACKET

COOKING TIME: 20 MIN | SERVES 4

INGREDIENTS:

- 2 russet potatoes, poked
- ½ tsp. salt
- Cooking spray
- 1 cup mild cheddar cheese, shredded
- 2 tsp. sour cream
- 1 garlic clove, minced
- ½ tsp. smoked paprika
- Chopped fresh chives (to garnish)
- Smoked paprika (to garnish)

DIRECTIONS:

1. Add salt and ½ cup water to the Ninja Foodi's insert and insert the reversible rack inside.
2. Place the potatoes in the reversible rack.
3. Put on the Pressure Lid and turn the pressure handle to the SEAL position.
4. Select Pressure Cook mode, set the pressure to High and cooking time to 10 minutes. Hit the START/STOP button to initiate cooking.
5. Once it's done, release the pressure quickly, then remove the lid.
6. Transfer the potatoes to a bowl and empty the pot.
7. Allow the potatoes to cool and make a slit on top of each potato.
8. Scoop out the flesh from the potato's skin and transfer the flesh to the Ninja Foodi's insert.
9. Mash the potatoes, then add garlic, sour cream and cheese, then mix well with the cooking liquid.
10. Mix well and cook on SEAR/SAUTE mode at High.
11. Divide this potato mash into the potato skins.
12. Place the stuffed potato jackets in the reversible rack.
13. Place the rack in the Ninja Foodi's insert and put on the crisping lid.
14. Cook on BROIL mode for 10 minutes.
15. Drizzle smoked paprika, chives and paprika over the potatoes.
16. Serve warm.

SAUCY STEWED VEGETABLES

COOKING TIME: 22 MIN | SERVES 6

INGREDIENTS:

Sauce
- 2 (14½-oz.) cans diced tomatoes with juice
- 1 yellow onion, diced
- 1 red bell pepper, seeded and diced
- 4 garlic cloves, minced
- 7 fresh basil leaves
- 3 tsp. olive oil

- ½ tsp. salt
- ¼ tsp. black pepper

Vegetables
- ½ Italian eggplant, sliced
- 3 vine-ripened tomatoes, sliced
- 1 yellow squash, sliced

- 1 zucchini, sliced
- Cooking spray
- Salt, to taste
- Black pepper, to taste
- 6 sprigs fresh thyme
- 1 tsp. basil leaves, torn
- 1 tsp. parsley, chopped

DIRECTIONS:

1. Add tomatoes, bell pepper, onion, basil, ½ cup water, black pepper, salt, olive oil, basil, and garlic to the Ninja Foodi's insert.
2. Put on the Pressure Lid and turn the pressure handle to the SEAL position.
3. Select Pressure Cook mode, set the pressure to High and cooking time to 2 minutes. Hit the START/STOP button to initiate cooking.
4. Once it's done, release the pressure quickly, then remove the lid.
5. Arrange the vegetable slices from the center of the pot, alternately in the Ninja Foodi's insert to make a spiral,
6. Drizzle black pepper, salt and thyme and put on the crisping lid
7. Cook on AIR CRISP mode at 390 degrees F for 20 minutes.
8. Serve warm.

FARRO ARUGULA SALAD

COOKING TIME: 10 MIN | SERVES 6

INGREDIENTS:

- 1 cup farro
- 2 fennel bulbs, halved, cored, and diced
- 2 fennel fronds, chopped
- 1 tsp. fennel seeds
- Zest and juice of 1 lemon
- 1 tsp. salt
- 2 tsp. olive oil
- 5 oz. arugula leaves

DIRECTIONS:

1. Add farro, 1 ¾ cups water, salt, lemon zest, fennel seeds and half the fennel to the Ninja Foodi's insert.
2. Put on the Pressure Lid and turn the pressure handle to the SEAL position.
3. Select Pressure Cook mode, set the pressure to High and cooking time to 10 minutes. Hit the START/STOP button to initiate cooking.
4. Once it's done, release the pressure naturally, then remove the lid.
5. Stir in fennel fronds, olive oil, salt, and arugula, then mix well.
6. Serve warm.

RED BEANS WITH WHITE RICE

COOKING TIME: 46 MIN | SERVES 4

INGREDIENTS:

RICE:
- 2 cups short-grain white rice, rinsed
- ½ tsp. salt

BEANS:
- 3 tsp. vegetable oil
- 3 celery stalks, chopped

- 1 medium yellow onion, diced
- 1 green bell pepper, seeded and diced
- 3 garlic cloves, minced
- 5 sprigs fresh thyme
- 2 dried bay leaves
- 3 tsp. Cajun seasoning
- 1 smoked ham hock

- 1-lb. dried red kidney beans
- 1 tsp. salt
- Fresh thyme leaves (to garnish)
- Black pepper (to garnish)

DIRECTIONS:

1. Add 2 cups water and rice to the Ninja Foodi's insert.
2. Put on the Pressure Lid and turn the pressure handle to the SEAL position.
3. Select Pressure Cook mode, set the pressure to High and cooking time to 3 minutes. Hit the START/STOP button to initiate cooking.
4. Once it's done, release the pressure naturally, then remove the lid.
5. Transfer the rice to a bowl and empty the pot.
6. Add oil, onion, bell pepper and celery to the Ninja Foodi's insert.
7. Sauté on SEAR/SAUTE mode at high for 6 minutes.
8. Stir in Cajun seasoning, bay leaves, thyme and garlic then sauté for 3 minutes.
9. Add 4 cups of water, kidney beans, and ham hock.
10. Put on the Pressure Lid and turn the pressure handle to the SEAL position.
11. Select Pressure Cook mode set the pressure to High and cooking time to 30 minutes. Hit the START/STOP button to initiate cooking.
12. Once it's done, release the pressure naturally, then remove the lid.
13. Stir in salt and divide the bean mixture into the serving bowls.
14. Add rice to the beans and garnish with pepper and thyme.
15. Serve warm.

ROASTED SQUASH MEDLEY

COOKING TIME: 25 MIN | SERVES 4

INGREDIENTS:

- 2 zucchinis, cut into rounds
- 2 yellow summer squash, cut into rounds
- ½ cup fresh parsley leaves
- 3 tsp. vegetable oil
- Zest of 1 lemon
- 2 tsp. salt
- ½ tsp. black pepper

DIRECTIONS:

1. Toss oil, zucchini, lemon zest, parsley, squash, black pepper and salt in a bowl.
2. Spread the squash mixture in the Ninja crisping basket and insert it into the Ninja Foodi's insert.
3. Put on the crisping lid and cook on AIR CRISP mode for 25 minutes at 390 degrees F.
4. Serve warm.

MAPLE DIPPED CARROTS

COOKING TIME: 29 MIN | SERVES 6

INGREDIENTS:

- 2 tsp. butter, unsalted
- 1 tsp. cumin (ground)
- 2 lbs. carrots, cut into 2" pieces
- ½ cup orange juice
- ¼ cup maple syrup
- 1 tsp. salt

DIRECTIONS:

1. Sauté cumin with butter in the Ninja Foodi's insert on SEAR/SAUE mode for 6 minutes.
2. Stir in orange juice and carrots then toss well.
3. Put on the Pressure Lid and turn the pressure handle to the SEAL position.
4. Select Pressure Cook mode, set the pressure to High and cooking time to 3 minutes. Hit the START/STOP button to initiate cooking.
5. Once it's done, release the pressure quickly, then remove the lid.
6. Add salt and maple syrup the put on the crisping lid.
7. Cook on AIR CRISP mode at 390 degrees F for 20 minutes.
8. Mix well and serve warm.

FRENCH HERBED BREAD STUFFING

COOKING TIME: 48 MIN | SERVES 6

INGREDIENTS:

- 1 loaf French bread, cut into cubes
- 4 tsp. butter, unsalted
- 1 yellow onion, diced
- 3 celery ribs, diced
- 1½ cups chicken stock
- 1 large egg, beaten
- 2 tsp. salt
- 1 tsp. black pepper
- 1 tsp. thyme leaves, minced
- 4 fresh sage leaves, minced
- Minced fresh parsley (to garnish)
- Fresh thyme leaves (to garnish)

DIRECTIONS:

1. Add the bread cubes to the Ninja crisping basket and insert them into the Ninja Foodi's insert.
2. Put on the crisping lid and cook DEHYDRATE mode for 15 minutes at 195 degrees F.
3. Transfer bread to a bowl and empty the pot.
4. Add butter to the Ninja Foodi's insert on SEAR/SAUTE mode at High for 5 minutes.
5. Stir in celery and onion then sauté for 8 minutes.
6. Add crispy bread cubes, sage and thyme.
7. Beat egg with black pepper, salt, and stock in a bowl.
8. Pour the prepared egg mixture over the bread cubes.
9. Put on the crisping lid and cook on BAKE/ROAST mode for 20 minutes at 375 degrees F.
10. Garnish with thyme and parsley.
11. Serve warm.

SPICED BEETS PICKLE

COOKING TIME: 1 MIN | SERVES 4 pints

INGREDIENTS:

- 8 beets, peeled, and cut into 8 chunks
- 2 cups apple cider vinegar
- 1 cup sugar
- 12 whole cloves
- 6 allspice berries
- 6 cardamom pods
- 1 cinnamon stick
- 2 tsp. salt
- 1 tsp. black peppercorns

DIRECTIONS:

1. Add peppercorns, salt, cinnamon stick, cardamom, allspice, cloves, sugar, vinegar and beets to the Ninja Foodi's insert.
2. Pour enough water to cover the beets and mix gently.
3. Put on the Pressure Lid and turn the pressure handle to the SEAL position.
4. Select Pressure Cook mode, set the pressure to High and cooking time to 1 minutes. Hit the START/STOP button to initiate cooking.
5. Once it's done, release the pressure quickly, then remove the lid.
6. Allow the beets to cool with the cooking liquid for 3 hours.
7. Discard the whole spices from the pickle and transfer the beets along with the liquid to 4 (1 pint) jars.
8. Seal the lid and refrigerate.

SAFFRON PILAF

COOKING TIME: 24 MIN | SERVES 4

INGREDIENTS:

- 3 tsp. vegetable oil
- ½ yellow onion, diced
- 1 garlic clove, minced
- 1 pinch of saffron threads
- ½ tsp. dried orange peel
- 2 cups basmati rice
- 2 cups chicken stock
- 1 (10-oz.) package frozen mixed vegetables
- ½ tsp. salt
- Sliced scallions (to garnish)
- sweet paprika (to garnish)
- Flat-leaf parsley (to garnish)

DIRECTIONS:

1. Preheat oil in the Ninja Foodi's insert on SEAR/SAUTE mode at High for 5 minutes.
2. Stir in garlic, onion, orange peel and saffron then sauté for 4 minutes.
3. Add rice and sauté for 4 minutes then pour in stock.
4. Put on the Pressure Lid and turn the pressure handle to the SEAL position.
5. Select Pressure Cook mode, set the pressure to High and cooking time to 3 minutes. Hit the START/STOP button to initiate cooking.
6. Once it's done, release the pressure naturally, then remove the lid.
7. Stir in mixed vegetables and put on the crisping lid.
8. Cook on AIR CRISP mode for 8 minutes at 390 degrees F.
9. Garnish with scallions, parsley and paprika.
10. Serve warm.

JALAPEÑO BRUSSELS SPROUTS

COOKING TIME: 23 MIN | SERVES 6

INGREDIENTS:

- 3 tsp. vegetable oil
- 2 lbs. Brussels sprouts, trimmed and scored
- 2 tsp. salt
- ½ tsp. black pepper
- 3 tsp. light brown sugar
- 2 tsp. fish sauce
- ¼ cup pickled jalapeños
- ¼ cup jalapenos pickling liquid
- Juice of 1 lime

DIRECTIONS:

1. Toss brussels sprouts with oil, black pepper and salt in a bowl.
2. Place the crisping basket in the Ninja Foodi's insert and spread the brussels sprouts to the basket.
3. Put on the crisping lid and cook on AIR CRSIP mode for 20 minutes at 390 degrees F.
4. Remove the basket and transfer the brussels sprouts to the Ninja Foodi's insert.
5. Stir in brown sugar, jalapenos, pickling liquid and fish sauce.
6. Switch the Ninja Foodi to SEAR/SAUTE at High for 3 minutes.
7. Stir in lime juice, then mix well.
8. Serve warm.

LEMONY GREEN BEANS

COOKING TIME: 27 MIN | SERVES 4

INGREDIENTS:

- 12 oz. fresh green beans, trimmed
- 1 tsp. vegetable oil
- ¼ tsp. salt
- Zest of 1 lemon
- 1 tsp. fresh dill, chopped

DIRECTIONS:

1. Mix beans, salt and oil in a bowl and spread them in the Ninja crisping basket.
2. Place the basket in the Ninja Foodi's insert and put on the crisping lid.
3. Cook on AIR CRISP mode for 15 minutes at 390 degrees F.
4. Drizzle dill and lemon zest over the beans after 12 minutes, then resume cooking.
5. Serve warm.

VEGETABLE FRIED RICE

COOKING TIME: 20 MIN | SERVES 6

INGREDIENTS:

- 2 cups short-grain white rice, rinsed
- 2 tsp. soy sauce
- 1 tsp. oyster sauce
- 1 tsp. sugar
- 1 tsp. black pepper
- ½ tsp. salt
- ¼ cup vegetable oil

- 2 large eggs, beaten
- 4 garlic cloves, minced
- 1 (10-oz.) package mixed frozen vegetables
- 3 scallions, trimmed and sliced

DIRECTIONS:

1. Add 2 cups of water and rice to the Ninja Foodi's insert.
2. Put on the Pressure Lid and turn the pressure handle to the SEAL position.
3. Select Pressure Cook mode, set the pressure to High and cooking time to 3 minutes. Hit the START/STOP button to initiate cooking.
4. Once it's done, release the pressure naturally, then remove the lid.
5. Transfer the cooked white rice to a bowl and allow them to cool.
6. Mix soy sauce, salt, black pepper, sugar, and oyster sauce in a small bowl.
7. Add oil to the Ninja Foodi's insert and heat on SEAR/SAUTE mode for 2 minutes.
8. Stir in eggs and sauté for 2 minutes.
9. Add garlic and sauté for 3 minutes then stir in rice.
10. Cook for 3 minutes then pour in soy sauce mixture. Cook for 2 minutes until liquid is absorbed
11. Make a small well with a spoon at the center of the rice and stir in vegetables.
12. Put on the crisping and cook AIR CRISP mode for 5 minutes at 390 degrees F.
13. Garnish with scallions.
14. Serve warm.

SPANISH RED QUINOA

COOKING TIME: 2 MIN | SERVES 6

INGREDIENTS:

- 1 cup white quinoa, rinsed
- 1 (14-oz.) can diced tomatoes with juice
- 2 garlic cloves, minced
- 1 tsp. cumin (ground)
- ½ tsp. chili powder
- ½ tsp. salt
- 1 tsp. butter, unsalted

DIRECTIONS:

1. Add butter, ½ cup water, salt, chili powder, cumin, garlic, tomatoes and their juice, and quinoa to the Ninja Foodi's insert.
2. Put on the Pressure Lid and turn the pressure handle to the SEAL position.
3. Select Pressure Cook mode, set the pressure to High and cooking time to 2 minutes. Hit the START/STOP button to initiate cooking.
4. Once it's done, release the pressure naturally, then remove the lid.
5. Fluff the cooked quinoa gently with a fork and serve.

CRUNCHY TURMERIC RICE

COOKING TIME: 21 MIN | SERVES 4

INGREDIENTS:

- 2 cups basmati rice
- 1 tsp. turmeric (ground)
- 1 tsp. salt
- 4 tsp. butter, unsalted

DIRECTIONS:

1. Add rice, turmeric, 2 cups water and salt to the Ninja Foodi's insert.
2. Put on the Pressure Lid and turn the pressure handle to the SEAL position.
3. Select Pressure Cook mode, set the pressure to High and cooking time to 3 minutes. Hit the START/STOP button to initiate cooking.
4. Once it's done, release the pressure naturally, then remove the lid.
5. Make a small well with a spoon at the center of the rice and drizzle 2 tbsp butter.
6. Switch the Ninja Foodi to SEAR/SAUTE mode and sauté for 8 minutes.
7. Put on the Crisping lid and cook on BROIL mode for 10 minutes.
8. Serve warm.

TOMATO & BULGUR SALAD

COOKING TIME: 6 MIN | SERVES 6

INGREDIENTS:

- 4 tsp. vegetable oil
- ½ tsp. cumin (ground)
- 1 cup whole-grain red bulgur
- 1 tsp. salt
- Zest and juice of ½ lemon
- 2 ripe plum tomatoes, halved, seeded, and diced
- 1 cucumber, seeded and diced
- 1 tsp. fresh mint, chopped
- 1 tsp. parsley, chopped
- Ground sumac (to garnish)
- Flat-leaf parsley (to garnish)

DIRECTIONS:

1. Add 3 tbsp oil in the Ninja Foodi's insert and heat on SEAR/SAUTE mode at high.
2. Stir in bulgur and cumin, then sauté for 3 minutes.
3. Add 2 cups water and ½ tsp. salt then mix gently.
4. Put on the Pressure Lid and turn the pressure handle to the SEAL position.
5. Select Pressure Cook mode, set the pressure to High and cooking time to 3 minutes. Hit the START/STOP button to initiate cooking.
6. Once it's done, release the pressure quickly, then remove the lid.
7. Add bulgur, remaining olive oil, and half of the lemon juice
8. Mix well and transfer the bulgur to a bowl.
9. Toss tomatoes with parsley, cucumber, mint, lemon juice, salt, lemon zest, parsley, and sumac in a bowl.
10. Mix the tabbouleh with tomatoes mixture in a bowl.
11. Serve.

BUTTERY COUSCOUS

COOKING TIME: 1 MIN | SERVES 4

INGREDIENTS:

- Cooking spray
- 1 cup couscous
- 2 tsp. butter, unsalted

DIRECTIONS:

1. Add butter 1 ½ cup water and couscous to the Ninja Foodi's insert.
2. Put on the Pressure Lid and turn the pressure handle to the SEAL position.
3. Select Pressure Cook mode, set the pressure to High and cooking time to 1 minute. Hit the START/STOP button to initiate cooking.
4. Once it's done, release the pressure naturally, then remove the lid.
5. Fluff the cooked quinoa gently with a fork and serve warm.

HERBED RISOTTO

COOKING TIME: 21 MIN | SERVES 4

INGREDIENTS:

- 4 tsp. butter, unsalted
- ½ yellow onion, diced
- 2 garlic cloves, minced
- 1 shallot, minced
- 1 cup arborio rice
- 1 cup dry white wine
- 2 cups Chicken stock
- 2 tsp. salt
- 1 cup Parmesan cheese, grated
- Finely chopped fresh chives (to garnish)
- Flat-leaf parsley (to garnish)

DIRECTIONS:

1. Melt butter in the Ninja Foodi's insert on SEAR/SAUTE mode at high.
2. Stir in shallots, garlic and onion, then sauté for 4 minutes.
3. Add rice and sauté for 4 minutes, then add wine and cook for 2 minutes.
4. Stir in stock and salt then mix gently.
5. Put on the Pressure Lid and turn the pressure handle to the SEAL position.
6. Select Pressure Cook mode, set the pressure to High and cooking time to 6 minutes. Hit the START/STOP button to initiate cooking.
7. Once it's done, release the pressure quickly, then remove the lid.
8. Switch the Ninja Foodi to the SEAR/SAUTE mode at high.
9. Add parmesan cheese and cook for 5 minutes.
10. Garnish with cheese and fresh herbs.
11. Serve warm.

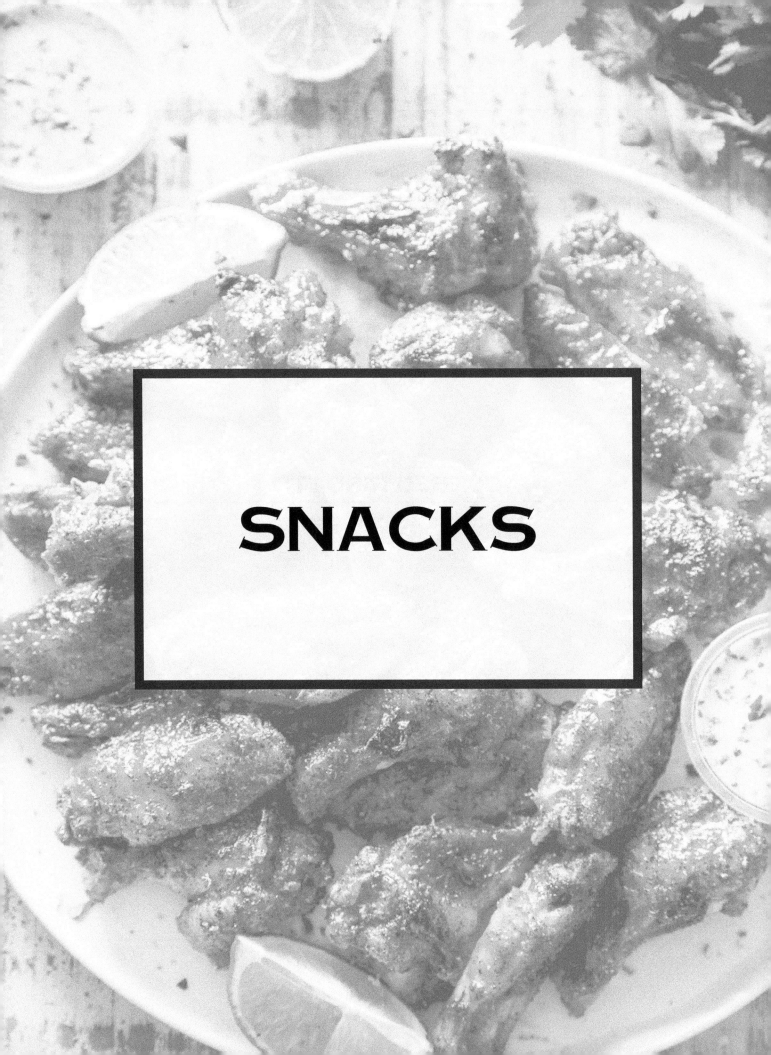

SNACKS

GARLIC FLATBREAD

COOKING TIME: 8 MIN | SERVES 10

INGREDIENTS:

- 1 tube of prepared pizza dough
- 1/2 cup butter
- 1 tsp. garlic
- 1 sprinkle of Italian seasoning
- 2 cups mozzarella cheese, shredded

DIRECTIONS:

1. Cut the pizza dough into 1-inch rounds and spread each into a six-inch diameter round.
2. Mix butter with herbs and garlic in a bowl and brush over the dough rounds.
3. Set the dough in the Ninja crisping basket and return the basket to the Ninja Foodi's insert.
4. Put on the crisping lid and cook AIR CRISP mode for 4 minutes.
5. Drizzle cheese and toppings on top.
6. Put on the crisping lid and cook AIR CRISP mode for 4 minutes.
7. Serve warm.

SPICY CHICKEN WINGS

COOKING TIME: 42 MIN | SERVES 2

INGREDIENTS:

- 1½ cups Frank's hot sauce
- 6 whole chicken wings, cut into flats and drumettes
- ½ tsp. salt
- Blue cheese dressing (to garnish)

DIRECTIONS:

1. Add 1 cup water and ½ cup hot sauce to the Ninja Foodi's insert.
2. Place the wings in the Ninja crisping basket and insert in the Ninja Foodi's insert.
3. Put on the Pressure Lid and turn the pressure handle to the SEAL position.
4. Select Pressure Cook mode, set the pressure to High and cooking time to 2 minutes. Hit the START/STOP button to initiate cooking.
5. Once it's done, release the pressure quickly, then remove the lid.
6. Drizzle salt over the wings and put on the crisping lid.
7. Cook on AIR CRISP mode at 390 degrees for 40 minutes.
8. Remove the basket from the Ninja Foodi's insert and transfer the wings to a bowl.
9. Add 1 cup hot sauce and toss well.
10. Garnish with blue cheese dressing.

TANGY WING SAUCE

COOKING TIME: 7 MIN | SERVES 1 CUP

INGREDIENTS:

- 4 tsp. butter, unsalted
- 6 oz. fresh blackberries
- 2 serrano chiles, chopped
- 1 tsp. black pepper

DIRECTIONS:

1. Add ½ cup water, black pepper, chiles, blackberries, and butter to the Ninja Foodi's insert.
2. Put on the Pressure Lid and turn the pressure handle to the SEAL position.
3. Select Pressure Cook mode, set the pressure to High and cooking time to 2 minutes. Hit the START/STOP button to initiate cooking.
4. Once it's done, release the pressure quickly, then remove the lid.
5. Mash the berries mixture using a potato masher, then switch the Ninja foodi to SEAR/SAUTE mode.
6. Cook the sauce for 6 minutes until it thickens.
7. Strain the blackberry mixture through a fine sieve into a bowl.
8. Allow the blackberry sauce to cool.
9. Serve.

MINI CRESCENT ROLLS

COOKING TIME: 16 MIN | SERVES 24

INGREDIENTS:

- 1 can (8 oz) refrigerated crescent rolls
- 24 mini sausages

DIRECTIONS:

1. Layer the Ninja Crisping Basket with 8-inch round parchment paper.
2. Spread the crescent on the working surface, cut it into 8 triangles, then slice each triangle into 3 triangles.
3. Place a mini sausage on one corner of each triangle and roll the triangles to wrap the sausage.
4. Set 12 of the wrapped rolls in the Ninja Foodi's insert and place it in the Ninja Foodi's insert.
5. Put on the crisping lid and cook on AIR CRISP mode at 325 °F for 8 minutes.
6. Flip the mini dogs once cooked halfway through, then resume the cooking.
7. Cook the remaining crescent dogs in the same manner.
8. Serve warm.

CHICKPEA HUMMUS

COOKING TIME: 30 MIN | SERVES 6 CUPS

INGREDIENTS:

- 1 lb. dried chickpeas
- 4 tsp. cumin seeds
- Zest of 1 lemon and
- Juice of 2 lemons
- ¾ cup tahini
- 1 cup olive oil
- 1 tbsp. toasted sesame oil

- 2 garlic cloves, minced
- 2 tsp. salt
- Pita bread (to serve)
- Vegetable sticks (to serve)

DIRECTIONS:

1. Add chickpeas, 5 cups water, lemon zest, and half of the cumin seeds to the Ninja Foodi's insert.
2. Put on the Pressure Lid and turn the pressure handle to the SEAL position.
3. Select Pressure Cook mode, set the pressure to High and cooking time to 30 minutes. Hit the START/STOP button to initiate cooking.
4. Once it's done, release the pressure naturally, then remove the lid.
5. Drain the cooked chickpeas and return to the Ninja Foodi's insert.
6. Add tahini, cumin seeds, garlic, salt, lemon juice, sesame oil, and olive.
7. Mix well and mash the chickpeas using a potato masher.
8. If the hummus is too thick, then add a cup of water.
9. Mix well and serve with pita bread and vegetable sticks.

CRISPY BACON WRAPPED HALLOUMI

COOKING TIME: 10 MIN | SERVES 12

INGREDIENTS:

- 6 streaky bacon rashers, cut in half
- 1 block halloumi
- Cooking spray

DIRECTIONS:

1. Slice the halloumi in half and cut each half into six equal-sized pieces.
2. Spread ½ a bacon rasher on the working surface and place a halloumi slice on top.
3. Wrap the rasher around the halloumi and continue the same with the remaining bacon and halloumi.
4. Place the wrapped halloumi in the Ninja Crisping Basket and spray them with cooking spray.
5. Transfer the Ninja Crisping Basket to the Ninja Foodi's insert and put on the crisping lid.
6. Cook on AIR CRISP mode at 335 °F for 10 minutes.
7. Serve warm.

CRUSTED JALAPEÑO POPPERS

COOKING TIME: 20 MIN | SERVES 24

INGREDIENTS:

- 1½ cups breadcrumbs
- 3 large eggs
- 1 (8-oz.) package cream cheese
- 1 (26-oz.) can pickled jalapeños, drained and halved
- Cooking spray

DIRECTIONS:

1. Spread breadcrumbs in one medium bowl and beat eggs in another bowl.
2. Stuff the jalapenos with cream cheese, then dip them in the egg and coat with breadcrumbs.
3. Place 9 coated jalapenos to the Ninja Crisping Basket and spray them with cooking spray.
4. Insert the Ninja Crisping Basket into Ninja Foodi's insert and cook on AIR CRISP mode at 390 °F for 10 minutes.
5. Cook the remaining jalapeno poppers in the same manner.
6. Serve warm.

CHICKEN CHEESE TAQUITOS

COOKING TIME: 15 MIN | SERVES 6

INGREDIENTS:

- 1½ cups cooked chicken, shredded
- 1½ cups Mexican-style cheese, shredded
- ¼ cup salsa
- 6 (8-inch) flour tortillas
- Cooking spray
- Sour cream (to serve)
- Salsa (to serve)
- Nacho cheese (to serve)

DIRECTIONS:

1. Mix chicken with salsa and cheese in a medium bowl, then mash a little to mix well.
2. Shape ¼ cup of the chicken cheese mixture into a log.
3. Place a tortilla on the working surface and top it with one chicken log.
4. Roll the tortilla and repeat the same with the remaining tortilla and chicken mixture.
5. Place the chicken rolls in the Ninja Crisping Basket and insert it into the Ninja Foodi's insert.
6. Spray the rolls with cooking spray and put on the crisping lid.
7. Cook on AIR CRISP mode at 390 °F for 15 minutes.
8. Flip the taquitos after 5 minutes and resume cooking.
9. Garnish with salsa, cheese, and sour cream.
10. Serve warm.

POTATO PAPAS BRAVAS

COOKING TIME: 31 MIN | SERVES 4

INGREDIENTS:

- 2 tbsp. butter, unsalted
- 2 tsp. sweet paprika
- 1 tsp. hot smoked paprika
- 1½ cups canned tomato sauce
- 1 tbsp. fresh oregano, minced
- 1 tbsp. sugar
- 1 tbsp. hot sauce
- ½ tsp. onion powder
- ¼ tsp. garlic powder
- 1 tsp. salt
- 1½ lbs. baby yellow potatoes
- 2 tbsp. vegetable oil

DIRECTIONS:

1. Add paprika and butter to the Ninja Foodi's insert and sauté on SEAR/SAUTE mode at High for 3 minutes.
2. Stir in sugar, oregano, tomato sauce, hot sauce, garlic powder, onion powder, and ½ tsp salt.
3. Mix and cook for 3 minutes, then pour the sauce into a bowl.
4. Toss potatoes with ½ tsp salt and oil in a bowl.
5. Spread the potatoes in the Ninja Crisping Basket and insert the basket in the Ninja Foodi's insert.
6. Put on the crisping basket and cook on AIR CRISP mode at 390 °F for 25 minutes.
7. Serve warm with prepared sauce.

LOADED NACHOS

COOKING TIME: 18 MIN | SERVES 4

INGREDIENTS:

- Cooking spray
- 8 (6-inch) corn tortillas, cut into six pieces
- Salt, to taste
- 8 oz. Mexican-style cheese, shredded
- Refried Black Beans (to serve)
- Sliced pickled jalapeños (to serve)
- Diced red onion (to serve)
- Pitted and sliced black olives (to serve)
- Guacamole (to serve)
- Sour cream (to serve)
- Cilantro (to serve)
- Salsa (to serve)

DIRECTIONS:

1. Grease the Ninja Crisping Basket with cooking spray and spread the tortillas in it.
2. Place the Ninja Crisping Basket in the Ninja Foodi's insert and put on the crisping lid.
3. Cook on AIR CRISP mode at 390 °F for 15 minutes.
4. Drizzle salt and cheese on top of the chips, then cover the crisping lid again.
5. Cook on BAKE/ROAST mode for 3 minutes at 375 °F.
6. Transfer the chips to a plate and top with refried beans, jalapenos, onion, guacamole, sour cream, cilantro, and salsa.
7. Serve warm.

BRAZILIAN CHEESE BREAD

COOKING TIME: 10 MIN | SERVES 8

INGREDIENTS:

- 1¼ cups whole milk
- 6 tbsp. vegetable oil
- 2 tsp. salt
- 4 cups tapioca flour
- 2 large eggs
- 1½ cups pecorino cheese, grated
- 1 cup packaged mozzarella, shredded
- Cooking spray

DIRECTIONS:

1. Add ½ water, oil, and milk to the Ninja Foodi's insert and cook for 5 minutes on SEAR/SAUTE mode at high.
2. Transfer the warm milk to a bowl and stir in tapioca flour, then mix well.
3. Beat in eggs, salt, and cheese, then mix well.
4. Grease the Ninja Foodi's insert with cooking spray and set the Ninja Crisping Basket inside.
5. Put on the crisping lid and preheat on BAKE/ROAST mode for 5 minutes at 375 °F.
6. Take a ¼ cup of the batter at a time and transfer it to the Ninja Crisping Basket. Add more batter to the basket in the same manner.
7. Put on the crisping lid and cook on BAKE/ROAST mode at 375 °F for 10 minutes.
8. Serve warm.

POTATO CRISPS

COOKING TIME: 18 MIN | SERVES 2

INGREDIENTS:

- 1 russet potato, peeled and paper-thin slices
- Cooking spray
- Salt, to taste

DIRECTIONS:

1. Soak the sliced potato in a bowl of water for 20 minutes, then drain.
2. Grease the Ninja Crisping Basket with cooking spray and spread the potato slices in the basket.
3. Put the basket in the Ninja Foodi's insert and cover the crisping lid.
4. Cook on AIR CRISP mode at 390 °F for 18 minutes.
5. Serve warm.

CRISPY MOZZARELLA STICKS

COOKING TIME: 10 MIN | SERVES 12

INGREDIENTS:

- ½ cup Italian style bread crumbs
- ½ cup panko bread crumbs
- ¼ cup parmesan cheese
- 1 tbsp. garlic powder
- 2 eggs
- 12 mozzarella cheese sticks, cut in half
- Cooking spray

DIRECTIONS:

1. Mix all the breadcrumbs with garlic powder and Parmesan cheese in a bowl.
2. Beat eggs in another bowl and dip all the mozzarella sticks in the eggs.
3. Coat the mozzarella sticks with the breadcrumb's mixture.
4. Set the mozzarella sticks in the Ninja Crisping Basket and spray them with cooking spray.
5. Put on the crisping lid and cook on AIR CRISP mode at 360 °F for 10 minutes.
6. Serve warm.

ZESTY CORN COB

COOKING TIME: 10 MIN | SERVES 3

INGREDIENTS:

- 3 corn on the cobb, shucked
- Cooking spray
- 1 tbsp. lemon zest
- 2 tbsp. cilantro, chopped

DIRECTIONS:

1. Place the corn cobbs in the Ninja Crisping Basket and drizzle lemon zest over them.
2. Spray them with cook spray and transfer the basket to the Ninja Foodi's insert.
3. Put on the crisping lid and cook on AIR CRISP mode for 10 minutes.
4. Drizzle salt and cilantro over the crispy corn.
5. Serve warm.

ALMOND & PEANUT BUTTER DONUT BITES

COOKING TIME: 3 MIN | SERVES 3

INGREDIENTS:

- 2 cups almond meal
- 1/2 cup peanut butter
- 1/3 cup honey

DIRECTIONS:

1. Mix almond meal with peanut butter and honey in a bowl to make a dough.
2. Spread the dough into a thick sheet and cut donuts using a cookie cutter.
3. Place the donuts in the Ninja Crisping Basket and spray them with cooking spray.
4. Transfer the basket to the Ninja Foodi's insert and put on the crisping lid.
5. Cook on AIR CRISP mode for 3 minutes at 350 °F.
6. Serve.

THICK CUT POTATO FRIES

COOKING TIME: 40 MIN | SERVES 2

INGREDIENTS:

- 3 large russet potatoes
- 2 tsp. salt
- Cooking spray

DIRECTIONS:

1. Cut the potatoes into thick-cut fries and soak them in a bowl filled with water.
2. Add ½ cup water and potatoes to the Ninja Foodi's insert.
3. Put on the Pressure Lid and turn the pressure handle to the SEAL position.
4. Select Pressure Cook mode, set the pressure to High and cooking time to 0 minutes. Hit the START/STOP button to initiate cooking.
5. Once it's done, release the pressure quickly, then remove the lid and empty the pot.
6. Drain and spread the potatoes in the Ninja Crisping Basket and spray them with cooking spray.
7. Place the basket in the Ninja Foodi's insert and put on the crisping lid.
8. Cook on AIR CRISP mode for 10 minutes at 275 °F.
9. Switch the Ninja foodi to 400 °F and cook for 30 minutes on AIR CRISP mode.
10. Serve warm.

DESSERTS

RASPBERRY SCONES

COOKING TIME: 25 MIN | SERVES 6

INGREDIENTS:

Raspberry compote:
- ½ cup frozen raspberries
- Juice of 1 small orange
- 1 tsp cornflour
- ⅓ cup caster sugar
- ¼ cup water

Scones:
- 1 ⅓ cups plain flour

- 2 ¾ tbsp. caster sugar
- ⅓ tsp cardamom (ground)
- 1 tsp baking powder
- ½ tsp bicarbonate of soda
- ¼ tsp salt
- ⅓ cup cold butter
- Zest of 1 small orange
- 1 egg

- ⅓ cup sour cream
- ¼ cup frozen raspberries
- ⅓ cup white chocolate, chopped
- 1 tsp milk
- 1 tsp demerara sugar
- Whipped cream (to serve)

DIRECTIONS:

1. Make raspberry preserve first, add the raspberries, caster sugar, and water to the Ninja Foodi's insert.
2. Cook on SEAR/SAUTE mode at MD: HI for 5 minutes with occasional stirring.
3. Reduce its heat to MD: LO and stir in the cornflour and orange juice, then mix well.
4. Cook the raspberry mixture until it thickens, then transfer the preserve to a bowl.
5. Empty the Ninja Foodi's insert and grease the Ninja Crisping Basket with parchment paper
6. Mix flour with caster sugar, baking powder, cardamom, salt, orange zest, salt, and bicarbonate of soda in a mixing bowl.
7. Cut in butter and mix well to a crumbly mixture.
8. Beat in sour cream and egg, then mix until it makes a smooth mixture.
9. Stir in white chocolate and raspberries.
10. Knead the dough and cut the dough into six even wedges. Dip the scones in milk and coat with sugar.
11. Place the scones in the Ninja Crisping Basket and transfer them to the Ninja Foodi's insert.
12. Put on the crisping lid and cook on BAKE/ROAST mode at 350 °F for 20 minutes.
13. Once cooled, serve with preserve and cream.

CINNAMON ROLLS

COOKING TIME: 10 MIN | SERVES 16

INGREDIENTS:

- 1 (9-inch) refrigerated pie dough
- 3 tbsp. unsalted butter, melted
- ¼ cup packed light brown sugar
- 2 tsp. cinnamon (ground)
- ¼ tsp. salt
- Cooking spray

DIRECTIONS:

1. Mix brown sugar with cinnamon and salt in a bowl.
2. Unroll the pie dough and brush the top with butter.
3. Drizzle cinnamon sugar on top and roll the dough.
4. Cut the cinnamon roll into ½ inch thick pieces.
5. Place the cinnamon rolls in the Ninja Crisping Basket and spray them with cooking spray.
6. Transfer the basket to the Ninja Foodi's insert and put on the crisping lid.
7. Cook on BAKE/ROAST mode for 10 minutes at 375 °F.
8. Serve.

VANILLA CRÈME BRULEE

COOKING TIME: 14 MIN | SERVES 4

INGREDIENTS:

- 6 eggs, separated
- ⅓ cup caster sugar
- 2 ⅛ cups double cream
- 1 ½ tsp vanilla extract
- 1/4 tsp salt
- Demerara sugar (for topping)

DIRECTIONS:

1. Beat the 6 egg yolks with sugar in a bowl.
2. Mix cream with salt and vanilla in a bowl, then heat this mixture in the microwave for 1 minute.
3. Add egg mixture into the cream mixture while mixing continuously until evenly mixed.
4. Beat egg white in a mixer until fluffy then add them to the batter. Mix gently.
5. Divide the batter into six 6 oz. ramekins and cover them with aluminum foil.
6. Set a reversible rack in the Ninja Foodi's insert and pour 13 ½ oz water into the pot.
7. Place the ramekins in the rack.
8. Put on the Pressure Lid and turn the pressure handle to the SEAL position.
9. Select Pressure Cook mode, set the pressure to LO and cooking time to 13 minutes. Hit the START/STOP button to initiate cooking.
10. Once it's done, release the pressure naturally, then remove the lid.
11. Allow the ramekins to cool and refrigerate for 4 hours.
12. Garnish each ramekin with 1 tsp sugar and melt it with a kitchen torch.
13. Serve.

DARK CHOCOLATE PUDDING

COOKING TIME: 20 MIN | SERVES 4

INGREDIENTS:

- 2 eggs, whisked
- 2 tsp. butter, melted
- 1 cup dark chocolate, melted
- 16 oz. cream cheese
- 2 tbsp. sugar

DIRECTIONS:

1. Grease 4 ramekins with cooking spray.
2. Beat eggs, butter, dark chocolate, cream cheese, and sugar in a mixing bowl.
3. Divide the pudding into the prepared ramekins.
4. Set a reversible rack in the Ninja Foodi's insert and pour 2 cups of water into the pot.
5. Place the ramekins in the rack.
6. Put on the Pressure Lid and turn the pressure handle to the SEAL position.
7. Select Pressure Cook mode, set the pressure to High and cooking time to 20 minutes. Hit the START/STOP button to initiate cooking.
8. Once it's done, release the pressure naturally, then remove the lid.
9. Allow the ramekins to cool and refrigerate for 4 hours.
10. Serve.

CLASSIC CHEESECAKE

COOKING TIME: 68 MIN | SERVES 4

INGREDIENTS:

- 1½ cups graham crackers, crushed
- 4 tbsp. butter, melted
- 1 pinch of salt
- 4 (8-oz.) packages cream cheese
- 1 (8-oz.) container sour cream
- 1 cup of sugar
- 1 tsp. vanilla extract
- Zest of 1 lemon
- 5 large eggs

DIRECTIONS:

1. Mix graham crackers with salt and melted butter in a bowl.
2. Spread the crackers mixture in a 9-inch springform pan.
3. Place the pan in the reversible rack and transfer it to the Ninja Foodi's insert.
4. Put on the crisping lid and cook on BAKE/ROAST mode at 350 °F for 8 minutes.
5. Meanwhile, beat cream cheese with sugar, lemon zest, vanilla, eggs, and sour cream in a bowl until fluffy.
6. Divide this cream cheese filling in the baked crust, then cover it with a foil sheet.
7. Add 2 cups water to the Ninja Foodi's insert and transfer the pan to the reversible rack.
8. Put on the Pressure Lid and turn the pressure handle to the SEAL position.
9. Select Pressure Cook mode, set the pressure to High and cooking time to 60 minutes. Hit the START/STOP button to initiate cooking.
10. Once it's done, release the pressure naturally, then remove the lid.
11. Allow the cake to cool and refrigerate for 8 hours.
12. Slice and serve.

CHERRY TART

COOKING TIME: 25 MIN | SERVES 4

INGREDIENTS:

- 2 tbsp. butter, melted
- 1 cup milk
- 3 large eggs
- ⅓ cup granulated sugar
- 1 tsp. vanilla extract
- ½ cup all-purpose flour
- 1 cup cherries, pitted and halved
- Confectioners' sugar (to garnish)

DIRECTIONS:

1. Grease a 9-inch springform pan with oil.
2. Beat eggs, milk, sugar, 2 tbsp butter, and vanilla in a bowl.
3. Stir in flour, then mix until smooth.
4. Spread the prepared batter in the prepared pan.
5. Set the reversible rack inside the Ninja Foodi's insert and place the pan in the rack.
6. Put on the crisping lid and cook on BAKE/ROAST mode at 325 °F for 25 minutes.
7. Transfer to a wire rack and allow it to cool.
8. Garnish with confectioner's sugar.
9. Slice and serve.

COCONUT SPICED SPONGE CAKE

COOKING TIME: 29 MIN | SERVES 4

INGREDIENTS:

- 7 oz. butter
- 1 cup caster sugar
- 1 ⅔ cups self-rising flour
- ½ cup desiccated coconut
- 4 large eggs
- 2 tbsp cardamom powder
- 6 ½ tbsp coconut milk
- ¾ cup icing sugar

Coconut Cream Icing
- 1 cup double cream, cold
- 1 cup icing sugar
- 7 oz. butter
- 3 drops coconut essence
- 2 cups strawberries, sliced (to garnish)

DIRECTIONS:

1. Mix flour with coconut and cardamom powder in a bowl.
2. Beat butter with sugar in a mixer until fluffy.
3. Add the 4 eggs and continue beating for 2 minutes.
4. Stir in the flour mixture, then mix until smooth.
5. Divide the batter into two seven inches baking pans and place one pan in the Ninja Crisping Basket.
6. Place the basket in the Ninja Foodi's insert and put on the crisping lid.
7. Cook on BAKE/ROAST mode for 25 minutes at 350 °F.
8. Meanwhile, beat coconut milk with icing sugar in a bowl and heat for 2 minutes in the microwave.
9. Transfer the prepared cake to a wire rack and bake the other half of the batter in the same way.
10. Poke holes in both the cakes and pour the milk mixture over them.
11. To make the icing, beat butter, coconut essence and icing sugar in a mixer until creamy.
12. Whip double cream until it makes soft peaks. Fold into the icing mixture.
13. Place the first cake on a serving plate and spread half of the icing and strawberries over the top of the cake.
14. Place the second cake on top and ice with the rest of the icing mixture. Arrange the remaining strawberries on top of the cake.
15. Slice and serve.

BANANA GINGER BREAD

COOKING TIME: 20 MIN | SERVES 6

INGREDIENTS:

- 4 bananas, peeled and mashed
- Cooking spray
- ½ cup unsalted butter
- 1 (½-inch) knob ginger, peeled and minced
- ¾ cup light brown sugar
- ½ tsp. salt
- 2 large eggs
- ¾ cup pecans, chopped
- 2 cups all-purpose flour
- 1 tsp. baking soda

DIRECTIONS:

1. Mix bananas with butter, ginger, sugar, salt, and eggs in a bowl until smooth.
2. Stir in baking soda, pecans and flour, then mix until all dry ingredients are incorporated.
3. Grease the Ninja Foodi's insert with cooking spray and spread the batter in the Ninja Foodi's insert.
4. Put on the crisping lid and cook on BAKE/ROAST mode for 15 minutes at 375 °F.
5. Switch the Ninja foodi to the SEAR/SAUTE mode and cook for 5 minutes.
6. Garnish with cream cheese and salt.
7. Slice and serve.

LAYERED VANILLA CRÈME

COOKING TIME: 24 MIN | SERVES 8

INGREDIENTS:

- 1 ½ cups caster sugar, divided
- 1 ⅓ cup water
- 5 eggs
- 1/4 tsp salt
- 3 cups whole milk
- 1 tsp vanilla extract

DIRECTIONS:

1. Add 2 oz water and 7 oz sugar to the Ninja Foodi's insert and cook for 5 minutes on SEAR/SAUTE mode at High.
2. Mix well, and cook for 10 minutes while mixing after every 2 minutes.
3. Once caramelized, divide the caramel into 8 ramekins and keep them aside.
4. Beat eggs with remaining sugar and salt in a stand mixer on low speed for 5 minutes.
5. Stir in vanilla and milk, then mix well for 2 minutes.
6. Divide this milk mixture into the ramekins and cover with a cling film.
7. Set a reversible rack in the Ninja Foodi's insert and pour 8 ½ oz water into the pot.
8. Place the ramekins in the rack.
9. Put on the Pressure Lid and turn the pressure handle to the SEAL position.
10. Select Pressure Cook mode, set the pressure to High and cooking time to 9 minutes. Hit the START/STOP button to initiate cooking.
11. Once it's done, release the pressure naturally, then remove the lid.
12. Allow the ramekins to cool and refrigerate for 4 hours.
13. Serve.

CHOCOLATE COFFEE CAKE

COOKING TIME: 20 MIN | SERVES 4

INGREDIENTS:

- ½ cup unsalted butter, melted
- ½ cup unsweetened cocoa powder
- 4 oz. bittersweet chocolate, melted
- ¾ cup of sugar
- 1 tsp. coffee granules
- ¼ tsp. salt
- 3 large eggs
- Vanilla ice cream (to serve)

DIRECTIONS:

1. Layer a 9-inch springform pan with parchment paper and grease it with butter.
2. Beat chocolate with melted butter in a bowl.
3. Stir in instant coffee, cocoa powder, sugar, and salt, then mix well.
4. Spread this batter in the prepared pan.
5. Set the reversible rack inside the Ninja Foodi's insert and place the pan on the rack.
6. Put on the crisping lid and cook on BAKE/ROAST mode at 350 °F for 20 minutes.
7. Once the coffee cake is baked, allow it to cool, then transfer to a plate.
8. Best served with ice-cream.

BAKED CUSTARD DESSERT

COOKING TIME: 45 MIN | SERVES 6

INGREDIENTS:

- 1¼ cups sugar
- 2 cups whole milk
- 1 tsp. vanilla extract
- 4 large eggs
- ½ tsp. salt

DIRECTIONS:

1. Set a reversible wire rack in the Ninja Foodi's insert and place an 8-inch disposable pie pan on it.
2. Spread 1 cup sugar in the pan and cook on SEAR/SAUTE mode for 30 minutes at High.
3. Allow the molted sugar to cool and remove the rack.
4. Add vanilla, milk, and remaining sugar to the Ninja Foodi's insert.
5. Cook on SEAR/SAUTE mode at High for 4 minutes, then transfer to a bowl.
6. Beat eggs with salt and 1 tbsp hot milk in a bowl for 6 minutes.
7. Pour into the milk mixture and beat well. Transfer this mixture to the pie plate.
8. Add ½ cup water to the Ninja Foodi's insert, set the reversible rack inside, and place the pan over it.
9. Put on the Pressure Lid and turn the pressure handle to the SEAL position.
10. Select Pressure Cook mode, set the pressure to High and cooking time to 5 minutes. Hit the START/STOP button to initiate cooking.
11. Once it's done, release the pressure naturally, then remove the lid.
12. Allow the ramekins to cool and refrigerate for 4 hours.
13. Flip the pan onto a plate and serve.

CHOCOLATE CHIP COOKIES

COOKING TIME: 10 MIN | SERVES 8

INGREDIENTS:

- 4 tbsp. butter, unsalted
- ¼ cup packed light brown sugar
- 2 tbsp. granulated sugar
- ½ tsp. salt
- 1 large egg yolk
- ¼ tsp. vanilla extract
- ½ cup all-purpose flour
- ¼ tsp. baking soda
- ¼ cup semisweet chocolate chips
- Cooking spray

DIRECTIONS:

1. Beat sugar with butter and salt in a mixing bowl.
2. Stir in vanilla and egg yolk, then beat until smooth.
3. Add baking soda and flour, then mix well until smooth.
4. Fold in chocolate chips, then mix gently.
5. Divide the prepared dough into 8 pieces and shape them into cookies.
6. Layer a Ninja Crisping Basket with aluminum foil and set the cookies in the basket.
7. Spray them with cooking spray and set the basket in the Ninja Foodi's insert.
8. Put on the crisping lid and cook on BAKE/ROAST mode at 325 °F for 10 minutes.
9. Allow the cooking to cool and serve.

APPLE DOUGHNUTS

COOKING TIME: 10 MIN | SERVES 6

INGREDIENTS:

- ½ cup plus 2 tbsp. all-purpose flour
- ¼ cup granulated sugar
- 1 tsp. cinnamon (ground)
- ½ tsp. salt
- ¼ tsp. baking powder
- ¼ tsp. baking soda

- ¼ cup milk
- 1 large egg white
- 2 tbsp. apple juice
- 2 tbsp. vegetable oil
- Cooking spray
- 2 tbsp. apple cider vinegar

Glaze:
- ½ cup confectioners' sugar
- 2 tbsp. apple juice

DIRECTIONS:

1. Grease 6 doughnut molds with cooking spray.
2. Set a reversible rack inside the Ninja Foodi's insert, put on the crisping lid, and preheat for 5 minutes at BAKE/ROAST mode at 375 °F.
3. Mix milk with apple cider and all the wet ingredients in a mixing bowl.
4. Stir in the rest of the dry ingredients, then mix well until smooth.
5. Divide the batter into the doughnut molds and transfer them to Ninja Foodi's insert.
6. Cover with the crisping lid and cook on BAKE/ROAST mode for 10 minutes at 390 °F.
7. Meanwhile, beat apple juice with sugar in a bowl.
8. Drizzle the glaze over the doughnuts.
9. Allow them to cool, then serve.

CREAMY CARAMEL SAUCE

COOKING TIME: 90 MIN | SERVES 2

INGREDIENTS:

- 1 can (14oz.) sweetened condensed milk
- 1 cup cold water
- ½ tsp. baking soda
- 3 tbsp. warm water

DIRECTIONS:

1. Mix warm water with baking in a bowl and leave it for 1 minute.
2. Pour soda mixture and milk into a stainless-steel bowl and mix well.
3. Add cold water to the Ninja Foodi's insert and set the bowl in the water.
4. Put on the Pressure Lid and turn the pressure handle to the SEAL position.
5. Select Pressure Cook mode, set the pressure to High and cooking time to 90 minutes. Hit the START/STOP button to initiate cooking.
6. Once it's done, release the pressure naturally, then remove the lid.
7. Blend the cooked mixture with a hand blender until smooth.
8. Allow to cool and get thicker.
9. Serve.

APPLE PIE TARTLETS

COOKING TIME: 5 MIN | SERVES 6

INGREDIENTS:

- 6 tart shells, thawed
- 1 cup apple pie filling
- ½ tsp. cinnamon
- A dash nutmeg

DIRECTIONS:

1. Place the tart shell in the Ninja Foodi's insert, put on the crisping lid, and cook on AIR CRISP mode for 7 minutes.
2. Mix pie fillings with nutmeg and cinnamon in a bowl.
3. Divide the filling in the tart shells and return the shells to the Ninja Foodi's insert.
4. Put on the crisping lid and cook on AIR CRISP mode for 5 minutes. Serve.

COCOA BROWNIES

COOKING TIME: 18 MIN | SERVES 2

INGREDIENTS:

- ½ cup granulated sugar
- 1/3 cup cocoa powder
- ¼ cup all-purpose flour
- ¼ tsp. baking powder
- 1 pinch salt
- ¼ cup butter, melted
- 1 egg

DIRECTIONS:

1. Grease a round baking pan with cooking and set it inside the Ninja Foodi's insert.
2. Mix sugar, salt, baking powder, flour, and cocoa powder in a large bowl.
3. Beat egg with butter and pour into the flour mixture.
4. Mix well until smooth, then pour the brownie batter into the pan in the insert.
5. Put on the crisping lid and cook AIR CRISP mode for 18 minutes at 350 degrees F.
6. Allow the brownies to cool, then slice. Serve.

VANILLA GLAZED DONUTS

COOKING TIME: 4 MIN | SERVES 8

INGREDIENTS:

- 1 Grands biscuit
- 2 cups sugar, powdered
- ¼ cup milk
- 1 tsp. vanilla extract

DIRECTIONS:

1. Place the grand biscuit on the working surface and cut circles out of it using a cookie cutter.
2. Set the biscuit rounds in the Ninja Crisping basket and spray them with cooking spray.
3. Place the basket in the Ninja Foodi's insert and put on the crisping lid.
4. Cook on AIR CRISP mode for 4 minutes at 350 degrees F.
5. Meanwhile, beat milk with vanilla and powdered sugar in a bowl.
6. Dip one side of the air crisped donuts in the milk glaze, then place them glaze side up on a cooling rack and allow to cool. Serve.

CREAMY BAKED ESPRESSO POTS

COOKING TIME: 10 MIN | SERVES 6

INGREDIENTS:

- 1 cup heavy cream
- ½ cup milk
- 1 tsp. espresso grains
- ¾ cup chocolate chips
- 3 egg yolks
- ¼ cup of sugar
- 1 tsp. vanilla extract
- 1 pinch of salt
- Whipped cream (to garnish)

DIRECTIONS:

1. Mix milk with heavy cream in the Ninja Foodi's Insert and cook on SEAR/SAUTE mode at HI until the mixture bubbles.
2. Pour the milk mixture into a bowl and stir in espresso and chocolate chips.
3. Mix well until the chocolate is melted, then set it aside.
4. Beat egg yolks with sugar in a bowl until pale. Stir in vanilla and chocolate mixture.
5. Divide the chocolate mixture into 4 small jars and close their lids.
6. Add 1 cup water to the Ninja Foodi's insert and set the steamer basket inside.
7. Set the lidded jars in the steamer basket.
8. Put on the Pressure Lid and turn the pressure handle to the SEAL position.
9. Select Pressure Cook mode, set the pressure to High and cooking time to 5 minutes. Hit the START/STOP button to initiate cooking.
10. Once it's done, release the pressure naturally, then remove the lid.
11. Allow the jars to cool, then refrigerate for 4 hours.
12. Garnish with whipped cream.
13. Serve.

CRÈME DE MENTHE CHEESECAKE

COOKING TIME: 25 MIN | SERVES 12

INGREDIENTS:

- 2 cups (24 Oreos) chocolate Oreos, crushed
- ¼ cup salted butter, melted
- 2 cups cream cheese
- ½ cup sugar
- 2 eggs
- 2 tbsp. Crème de Menthe
- 1 tsp. mint extract
- 10 drops green food coloring
- 1 bar mint chocolate, grated (to garnish)

DIRECTIONS:

1. Blend oreos with melted butter in a blender or food processor and spread the mixture in a 9-in baking tin.
2. Beat cream cheese with egg, sugar, food color, crème de menthe, and mint extract in a mixer for 3 minutes.
3. Spread this mint cream cheese in the prepared crust in the pan.
4. Add 1 cup water to the Ninja Foodi's insert and set a rack inside.
5. Set the pan on the rack inside the pot.
6. Put on the Pressure Lid and turn the pressure handle to the SEAL position.
7. Select Pressure Cook mode set the pressure to High and cooking time to 25 minutes. Hit the START/STOP button to initiate cooking.
8. Once it's done, release the pressure naturally, then remove the lid.
9. Allow the cheesecake to cool. Top the cake with grated mint chocolate shavings.
10. Slice and serve.

CPSIA information can be obtained
at www.ICGtesting.com
Printed in the USA
BVHW061646131221
623925BV00012B/304